The Accidental cure*

The SECRET *Treatment your doctor will not tell you*
The true story of my recovery from
Multiple Sclerosis and Celiac Disease

*cure *n* 1 A method or course of medical treatment
2 Restoration of health

DEBBIE MCGRANN

The Accidental Cure © 2019 Debbie McGrann

All rights reserved. Printed in the United States of America. No part of this book may be used or reproduced in any manner whatsoever without written permission except in the case of quotations embodied in reviews or used for educational purposes.

DISCLAIMERS

Although the author and publisher have made every effort to ensure that the information in this book was correct at press time, the author and publisher do not assume and hereby disclaim any liability to any party for any loss, damage, or disruption caused by errors or omissions, whether such errors or omissions result from negligence, accident, or any other cause.

This book is not intended as a substitute for the medical advice of physicians. The reader should regularly consult a physician in matters relating to his/her health and particularly with respect to any symptoms that may require diagnosis or medical attention.

Editing by
Teresa Hamilton
Doc Wilson
Phillip Wizeman
Katherine Trezise

Book and Cover design by Francis Adams

ISBN 978-1-7337189-4-3

First Edition: November 2019

CONTENTS

Acknowledgments..5
Dedication..6
Why Did I Choose This Title?..7
Mission Statement..9
Introduction..12
Are You Ready to Be Well?..14
My List of Symptoms..17
Be Grateful for Who You Are...19

CHAPTER ONE *WHY I AM THE WAY I AM*......................21
    Life in Oklahoma
    Growing Up in Washington, DC
    Courage Under Fire
    A Childhood in Chaos
    My Career Path
    Family Changes

CHAPTER TWO *DISCOVERING MY DIAGNOSIS*.............45
    Early Symptoms
    Impact on My Family
    If MS is not Fatal, What's Killing Me?
    Symptoms Over Time
    My Pain Became My Information

CHAPTER THREE *I LEARNED TO ALWAYS BE PERSISTENT*...............69
    Marching Onward

CHAPTER FOUR *I WAS CHOSEN: "WHY ME?" "WHY NOT ME?"*............73
    Why?
    The Discovery Process

CHAPTER FIVE *BECOMING FEARLESS*..........................81
    New Year's Day 2008
    Mother's Day - A Critical, Impactful Decision

CHAPTER SIX *A MEASURE OF FAITH*............................89
    Faith
    Maintaining a Positive Mental State
    Reaction to Recovery
    Dream Big! Get Your Life Back!

CHAPTER SEVEN *THE ANSWER TO MY MEDICAL MYSTERY*..............107
    Meeting Dr. Fasano
    Conclusion
    Celiac Disease - An Introduction
    Prevalence of the Problem - The Leaky Gut Theory
    Recovery
    Support Groups

CHAPTER EIGHT *MY NEW NORMAL*..............119
    Communicating My New Life to Family and Friends
    Would Your Doctor Lie to You?

CHAPTER NINE *DRUGS OR NO DRUGS*..............127
    MS Drugs vs Gluten free Diet: What Would You Do?
    Are the Drugs and Bankruptcy Worth Dying For?
    Calculating the Cost
    Tysabri - A Case Study
    Death and Dividends: The Tysabri Debacle

CHAPTER TEN *EMBARKING ON A GLUTEN-FREE DIET*..............137
    Gluten-free Diet as the Cure for Celiac Disease
    Tips for Starting a Gluten-free Dietary Treatment
    General Foods to Eat When on a Gluten-free Diet

CHAPTER ELEVEN *THE FUTURE OF CELIAC DISEASE*..............143
    Why is Celiac Disease Increasing?
    Attention Deficit Hyperactivity Disorder (ADHD)
    Multiple Sclerosis (MS) and Celiac Disease
    Autism

CHAPTER TWELVE *LIVING LIFE TO ITS FULLEST*..............151
    Healthy, Wealthy & Wise
    What If?

List of 100 Autoimmune Diseases..............161

Epilogue..............169

References..............172

About the Author..............185

Acknowledgments

I would like to take this opportunity to thank those who have helped me make this book possible. The team at Imagination Press listened to my dream of this book and helped me turn my dream into reality. They believed in the project from the very first day. They valued my story, and knew it needed to be told in order to help others recover their health. Their advice and directions were what got us to the finish line. This is my opportunity to extend my sincere appreciation to Teresa Hamilton for managing what seemed to me, in the beginning, to be an overwhelming project. Her patience kept everything on track.

Many thanks to Doc Wilson, Phillip Wizeman, and Katherine Trezise for their expert editing. Thank you to Francis Adams for his layout and cover designs. These individuals provided me with valuable guidance, encouragement, and their professional skills in order to reach my goal.

Finally, I would like to thank the agents and staff in my Coldwell Banker real estate office. Their encouragement and kind words helped me more than they will ever know.

Dedication

This book is dedicated to my Grandparents and Parents.

My Aunts, Uncles, and Cousins
My Brother Jimmy, Sister Kathy and my other Sister Kathy
My Sisters-in-law, Brothers-in-law, Nieces and Nephews

My Children Jimmy, Jennifer and son-in-law Jason
My Grandchildren Ella, Avery and John

With special dedication to my Husband Jim:
We started life together in 1972, just the two of us
working together building our family and business, never realizing
what was in store for us.
With my disability looming over us,
we tackled it head on and defeated it together, never giving up!

For better or worse, in sickness & health, for richer or poorer;

We live our vows each day.
Remember, the best is yet to come!

Forever & Ever. Amen.

Why Did I Choose This Title?

The Accidental Cure. From where did this title come? When I started thinking about my responsibility to tell my story in print, I thought about the fact that I had discovered my treatment plan completely by accident. No doctor had suggested this simple treatment to me. It was as if the information was a secret that had to be discovered by the patient. As I explain the chain of circumstances that revealed this secret information to me, I think you will come to fully understand the title.

I have received a lot of criticism from friends and readers of my previous writings regarding the use of the word "Cure." They have told me that – since I was not a doctor, and there was no cure for Multiple Sclerosis – I should be careful using that word. Also, they thought that I should not give false hope to Multiple Sclerosis patients by telling them that they can be cured. As a patient with Multiple Sclerosis who had seen many doctors over many years, none of whom had given me ANY hope of getting better, and knowing that I would have welcomed any hope of a cure that was founded on solid evidence, I knew that, like me, other patients would welcome knowing that there was at least a chance that they could get better.

Based on my extensive experience, there now is evidence that MS patients are getting better – even cured – when they follow the simple treatment that I discovered. However, doctors are not passing this information on to their patients.

> Let me remind you of the meaning of the noun **cure**:
> 1. A method or course of medical treatment.
> 2. Restoration of health.

Once you read my story, I am sure that you will agree that I am cured of MS, and that you, too, have a reasonable chance of restoring your health if you do what I did.

DEBBIE MCGRANN

Mission Statement

Inspire. Inform. Educate. Empower. Motivate.

I will use the true story of my recovery from Multiple Sclerosis as a way to bring awareness to Celiac Disease.

Inspire
My goal with this book is to inspire you to seek the answers you need for your health issues. I want to inspire you to be brave and question authority. I hope that my story is the inspiration that you need to live your best life. There is HOPE for your recovery just like my recovery. I do not fear that my words will offend someone because I have confidence that my words will inspire someone.

Inform
The purpose of this book is to inform readers of my recovery from MS and provide the information they need for their own recovery. I am convinced that my recovery would have been a lot sooner if I had been provided more information about treatment options. Information on MS, and other autoimmune diseases, is controlled by the drug companies to the doctors. The doctors are being manipulated. Are the drug companies providing information, advertising, or propaganda?

Patients must assume that their doctors, the MS Society, and other groups claiming to represent the patient's best interest, have been manipulated by the drug companies. This is due to the support that they receive from drug company donations and advertising fees. Therefore, the best hope for recovery is for the patient to seek out information from other sources. The information is there. I will provide as much as I can in this book. I am committed to continuing beyond this book to provide ongoing information and support.

Educate
Education does not end with diplomas. We must be lifetime learners. My life depended on what I could learn on my own about MS treatments. I did not need a college or medical degree to read medical articles on MS and discover for myself the treatment that would stop my disability from progressing and save my life. The information is out there, and it is free.

Empower
I want to empower you with confidence to think for yourself, ask questions, and seek answers. This is important in all areas of your life. We cannot rely on others to make it all better. Of course, we can accept help from others. However, we have to be the one in control.

Motivate
One of my favorite motivators is Zig Ziglar. I would encourage you to read as many of his writings as you can.

"Motivation is the spark that lights the fire of knowledge and fuels the engine of accomplishment. It maximizes and maintains MOMEMTUM"

Zig Ziglar

"Of course, motivation is not permanent. But then, neither is bathing; but it is something you should do on a daily basis."

Zig Ziglar

Take his advice. Find things that motivate you. I found motivation in different ways: music, sporting events, reading, church services, and socializing. Find the activities that motivate you. Motivation is the key to persistence. We need to motivate ourselves daily to lift our spirits and help us accomplish our goals.

Introduction

How did I, a 50-year-old woman with less than two years of college, think I could discover the cure for my Multiple Sclerosis? I knew that the doctors did not know what causes Multiple Sclerosis, nor did they know of a cure for Multiple Sclerosis, so, I knew as much (or as little) as they did. But I had some things the doctors didn't have:

TIME:
Multiple Sclerosis is a chronic, complex disease. Doctors do not have time to research an individual's symptoms to come up with proper treatments, especially if the treatment does not include drugs. I was firmly committed to spending as much time as necessary to find a cure for my Multiple Sclerosis.

MOTIVATION:
My motivation was pain - constant, debilitating pain - pain that was getting worse every day. I was running out of time. The doctors were focused on treating my pain symptoms, but I needed to find the source of the pain. I did not want to learn to live with the pain. I was motivated to get well and find a cure.

FAITH:
How strong was my faith? In whom did I have faith? At the beginning of my medical journey, my faith in my doctors was very strong. However, I learned that my faith in them was misplaced. I decided that, if I was going to get better any time soon, I had to take control of my cure.

I was not going to let *anything* stop me from finding the answers I needed, especially my fear of asking "stupid" questions. I began telling everyone I met that I had Multiple Sclerosis.

After my New Year's Day announcement that I would cure my Multiple Sclerosis, the answers to my medical problems started to come very quickly and in many forms: casual conversations, books, research, websites, consultations with doctors, etc. On Mother's Day of 2008 (only 18 weeks later!), I started the treatment that would cure my Multiple Sclerosis and my other health problems <u>without drugs of any kind.</u> Not one of my many doctors had ever suggested this simple cure to me.

Are You Ready to Be Well?

Are you ready to be well? That sounds like a funny question. However, in order to be well, sometimes we must have the courage to change what we have been doing. As patients, we must learn to take charge of our own recovery and health. The doctor's role should be that of a partner, not a repairman.

I never took the Multiple Sclerosis drugs that the doctors had advised me to take. I thought the side effects were too much of a risk. I did take a common drug for my osteoporosis and had a severe reaction to it. If all we do is take medicine and ignore our diet and lifestyle, we are wasting our doctor's time, wasting money, and jeopardizing our recovery. Are you sick and tired of being sick and tired? What changes are you ready to make?

In my case, I discovered that my diet must be gluten-free. The changes were difficult at first. But the diet got easier as my pain started to go away, and my health improved remarkably! I have Celiac Disease that had been undiagnosed since childhood. If you have an autoimmune disorder like Multiple Sclerosis, including fibromyalgia, lupus, osteoporosis, arthritis, diabetes, chronic fatigue, etc., you may also have undiagnosed Celiac Disease.

The doctors told me that damage to my immune system is what caused my Multiple Sclerosis. I have since learned that gluten is what damaged my immune system.

Here is a simple old-time formula for good health:

> "The best six doctors anywhere
> And no one can deny it
> Are sunshine, water, rest, and air
> Exercise and diet.
> These six will gladly you attend
> If only you are willing
> Your mind they'll ease
> Your will they'll mend
> And charge you not a shilling."
> **Wayne Fields**

Should we take medical advice from a poem? Well, have you ever heard a doctor say that those six recipes for health are bad for you?

I saw a post on Facebook of a friend from high school. She was asking, "Have you ever been in so much pain that the bedsheets caused more pain when they touched your skin?" She commented that her fibromyalgia was flaring up.

I responded to her post, "Yes." I had experienced that much pain. I told her about my MS and my recovery after going on a gluten-free diet. I told her that fibromyalgia patients were having similar success on the diet. I suggested that she should try the diet to help with her pain.

She responded back to me that she knew about the diet. She had tried it in the past and it was successful in helping with her pain and other symptoms. But, "I love bread and pasta so much!"

Why was she willing to keep suffering when she knew the

answer to her problem? Her pain couldn't have been that bad if she chose bread and pasta over eliminating her pain. Or, did she enjoy the attention? Having a disease like MS, fibromyalgia, or similar autoimmune diseases brings you attention and sympathy from family and friends. The more I share my story with other patients, the more people I meet who don't want to get better. Attention can be intoxicating to some people!

I would rather cure my pain than have the attention. I would rather have a job and work than be on disability.

The only question remaining, then, is this: Are you ready to change your behavior so you can start getting well?

My List of Symptoms

I experienced these symptoms throughout my illness. Are you suffering with any of these symptoms? If so, I am confident that the information in this book is likely to help you.

- Paleness
- Loss of muscle tone
- Loss of weight
- Low blood sugar (hypoglycemia)
- Vision problems
    - *Floaters and Flashers*
    - *Double vision*
- Numbness (starting in my feet and spreading to the rest of my body over time)
- Vertigo
- Fainting
- Low blood pressure (hypotension)
- Restless legs
- Pain
    - *Muscle pain*
    - *Bone pain*
- Hearing problems
    - *Pain in my ears*
    - *Ringing in my ears*
    - *Slushing sounds in my ears*
- Speech problems
    - *Confusion with words*
    - *Voice weakness*
    - *Slurring words*
- Lactose intolerance
- Chronic fatigue
- Brain fog
    - *Trouble remembering details*

- Hypersensitivity
    - *Sounds*
    - *Smells*
    - *Heat*
- Clumsiness
    - *Dropping items*
- Random burning sensations
- Random inching sensations
- Eczema
- Walking difficultly
    - *Heavy legs*
    - *Falling and tripping*
- ADHD
- Osteoporosis
- Pernicious Anemia (a Vitamin B-12 deficiency)
- Vitamin D deficiency
- Allergies
- MS

<u>NOTE:</u> You could have symptoms that are different from those that I experienced.

Be Grateful for Who You Are

On one of my many visits to have blood drawn for more testing, the nurse helping me made the comment, "I wish I was like you." I was lying down on the bed so that I wouldn't faint after the blood was drawn.

She looked like she was in her late 30s or early 40s. She was tall, and I would say stocky. I thought she was very pretty, professional, and very nice.

I asked her what she meant by that comment. She replied, "I wish I was tall and thin like you." I told her to look at my medical chart to see what they were testing me for, and what my diagnosis was. She reviewed the chart and said, "Never mind."

I asked her if she was in good health, and blood pressure good? "Yes." Did she have children? "Yes." Are they healthy? "Yes." "Then, you don't want to be like me," I said.

I smiled and told her to be grateful for who she was, and the blessings that she had. The moral: Never wish to be someone else if you do not fully know what they are going through.

TOUGHNESS

"Most of the important things in the world have been accomplished by people who have kept on trying when there seemed to be no hope at all."
Dale Carnegie

"Promise me you'll always remember: You're braver than you believe, and stronger than you seem, and smarter than you think."
Christopher Robin to Pooh - A.A.Milne

"Do not pray for an easy life, pray for the strength to endure a difficult one."
Bruce Lee

"Tough times never last, but tough people do!"
Dr. Robert H. Schuller

CHAPTER ONE

Why I Am the Way I Am

Life in Oklahoma

My family history consists of stories of hardship and poverty that were defeated by faith, courage, toughness, strength, and hard work.

My mother, Alberta Mae Carson (Mary Ann), was the youngest of five children born in the outskirts of Oklahoma City. Born in 1936 at the height of the Depression and the Great Dust Bowl, she was delivered on the kitchen table with the assistance of her father and a midwife – just like her older brother and sisters. Their family home, a wooden shack with a tin roof and a dirt floor, was located behind my mother's Aunt Lee Bush's house. Kids were not allowed in Aunt Lee's house because she did not like children.

Soon, things got more complicated and challenging when more relatives moved into the house. Aunt Kit remembers that the kids slept on the dirt floor, except my mother, who, as an infant, slept in a dresser drawer. They were literally "dirt poor" – with no electricity, no heat, and no indoor plumbing.

According to Aunt Kit, my grandmother and her friend Faye, did anything they could to make money – including cleaning houses and picking strawberries; in addition, they picked and cleaned turkeys for pennies a piece.

My grandfather was a carpenter with his father but was not a hardworking man. When President F.D. Roosevelt came into office during the Great Depression and the drought, he created the Works Progress Administration (WPA) to put people back to work. Under WPA, my grandfather worked in the stock yards as a butcher. This work sufficed until the drought worsened, and all the cattle either died or were butchered early. Soon, work in Oklahoma disappeared, and adults had little hope of a better life.

While they lived in Oklahoma, my mother's brother and sisters played outside with games like kick the can, mother may I, and dodge ball, as well as built stilts. At night, they enjoyed catching lightning bugs and keeping them in jars. The adults watched the kids play from their position on the porch as they themselves played dominoes and card games. For entertainment, the family watched adult women's softball league games at a nearby stadium. There was never money for ice cream, popcorn, or anything extra; however, the children were free to run and play with their friends.

Aunt Kit remembers: *In the fall, my dad and the other men hunted – bringing home lots of rabbits. It seemed that all we ate was rabbits. Mom skinned them, cleaned them, and hung them on the back porch – hoping that they would freeze so that they would be safe to eat. When mom fried them, they tasted like fried chicken. We also had a creek that had crawdads that we caught and ate. In addition, we sometimes fished for catfish, which we liked to eat. Furthermore, mom had a great garden that produced lots of okra, kale, collards, beans, and potatoes.*

My grandmother hated living in Oklahoma. She was from the North Carolina coastal town of Wilmington, where she had enjoyed living near the water, and had a huge variety of trees and flowers around her. She did not like the tumbleweed plants of Oklahoma. Of course, she was in Oklahoma during the Dust Bowl years when it would have been difficult to grow anything! Nevertheless, she did the best she could with what she had. She canned beans, tomatoes, pickles, etc. – storing them in the storm cellar. The violent storms of Oklahoma terrified her. She told me many stories of the lighting storms she had seen there. During the dust storms, she turned all the dishes upside-down on the table so that they would not be covered with dust; in addition, everyone had to cover their face with wet cloths when they went to the outhouse.

Saturday was a workday in which to prepare for Sunday because their church did not allow any activities on Sunday other than worship services. On Sundays, no one was allowed to read the newspaper, wear makeup, dance – not even cook. Therefore, the main activity for Saturday was preparing food for Sunday. If fried chicken was on the menu, grandmother went into the yard and caught three or four chickens, wrung their necks, and put them in hot scalding water; then, the older kids plucked the feathers. My grandmother then hung the chickens on the clothesline until she was ready to fry them. Sometimes, on the same day, she made homemade ice cream, cheese, cottage cheese, and sour cream.

There was no inside plumbing. The kids took a bath Saturday night in a huge steel tub. My grandmother washed the girls' hair and curled their hair in rags. Aunt Kit remembers how hard it was to sleep with rags in her hair, especially when sleeping on the hard dirt floor; but the kids did what they were told.

My grandmother raised her children in the church and taught them right from wrong. How they turned out later in life was each one's individual choice; however, she always wanted the best for her children. Aunt Kit remembers many times seeing her cry because she could not provide enough food for her family. There was no money for Christmas or birthday gifts. No wonder Washington, DC looked like paradise to my grandmother, although, in the end, it certainly did not turn out that way.

Like thousands of other families, my grandparents were driven out of Oklahoma because of the depression and the drought, which left few options for them. I once asked my grandmother why they moved to Washington, DC in view of the fact that many other families fled to California – just like in the book and movie, *The Grapes of Wrath*. She replied that she had family in Washington with whom they could live until they found a place of their own.

How to get to DC? My grandparents ran an ad in the newspaper offering to pay the expenses for anyone who would drive them to Washington, DC. A stranger with a small Model T drove them to DC. My grandfather sat up front, and my grandmother and the five children sat in the backseat. My mother, three years old, sat on my grandmother's lap. Since there were no interstate highways, they drove straight across, the country, eastward, and over the Appalachian Mountains. Aunt Kit recalled that it was a horrible trip, and that my Aunt Joann was carsick for most of the five-day trip.

When my grandmother told me about the trip to Washington, DC, she said that she was only allowed to take her sewing machine, a small radio, and her cast iron skillet (which I still have today). She said that the children were allowed to take only what they could carry. Aunt Kit was upset because she had to leave her pet chickens behind.

Growing Up in Washington, DC

When they arrived in Washington DC, Aunt Kit said that all of the kids hated it. They had always lived in the country, and now they were in downtown Washington, DC. What a shock: from one extreme to another. As bad as Oklahoma had been, they wanted to go back because their housing situation was no better. They moved into an apartment above a shoe store, which they shared with two other families – my grandmother's sisters, Bonnie and Helen, their husbands, and a total of six children. Each family had one bedroom, and they shared a kitchen. That meant two adults and three children per bedroom. In addition, my grandparents and their five children lived in another room – for a total of six adults and eleven children in one apartment. The bathroom was an outhouse in the alley, which was reached by going down the fire escape to the roof of the shoe store, and then down another flight of stairs to the alley. The children's playground was a small patch of concrete in the alley below the fire escape. They lived in the slums of Southwest Washington – some of the worst slums in the country! The city streets and the filthy Potomac river of Washington, DC were far different from the open fields and sparkling creeks of Oklahoma.

Shortly after arriving in DC, my mother had an accident that not only shaped the rest of her life, but also dramatically impacted her family. I heard this story often. Aunt Kit described it as follows:

"One day, Mary Ann (my mother), three or four years old, was going down the steps to the outhouse. Somehow, she lost her footing and fell two stories to the concrete of the alley, landing face down. I will always remember how her face looked as they came up the stairs with her. Her face was swollen and covered with blood. She was taken to the hospital. She had a fractured skull, a huge gash in her

forehead, a broken pelvis, and numerous other injuries. The doctors said she would not live through the night, but she did. Mom stayed with her in the hospital for months. I remember that mom used to take Mary Ann chocolate covered malt balls because she said that they would melt in her mouth, and she would not choke.

She was put in a body cast from her neck to the end of each foot. In addition, a pole was placed between her feet. She had to be carried everywhere. She was left with large scars on her forehead, and I always thought that her adult back problems came from this fall."

Aunt Kit and my grandmother told me that my mother's accident happened on a Friday the 13th. As children, we always lived within blocks of my grandparents' house. Every Friday the 13th, my grandmother called my mother and told her to stay in bed, and then came over to stay with us kids. Of course, my mother never stayed in bed, but my grandmother still came over to be with her and the rest of us.

Aunt Kit was about nine years old when it came time for the kids to start school in DC. My mother was too young for school and was still in her body cast. Aunt Kit remembers her teacher asking her if she was from *The Grapes of Wrath* or *Tobacco Road*. At the time, she did not know how much of an insult this was from her teacher. My Uncle told similar stories about being bullied by other students. He went to school in DC the same way he had in Oklahoma: in overalls and barefooted. The teachers and students called them "poor Okies," and made fun of the way they talked. School was not a haven for them.

Because of their conditions at home, they didn't have anywhere to study. Aunt Kit remembers her French teacher discussing her poor grade with her. This teacher somehow knew that Aunt Kit attended the local church. She called Aunt Kit a religious fanatic and told her to get out of the church or she was going to fail. Aunt Kit told her that the church did not have anything to do with her performance in school. The family did not have heat all the way through high school.

The family moved once again – this time to a house in Southwest DC. There was no electricity, no running water, and no bathroom – only a broken-down outhouse. All five of the kids shared the front room on the third floor. My mother had a bed because of her cast, and her brother and sisters slept on the floor. Because there was no heat, they slept in their coats. My grandmother brought them water at night; by morning it was frozen solid.

Because they lived near the Potomac River, the house was swarming with huge rats, cockroaches, and bed bugs. At night, the rats chewed on my mother's cast.

> **Imagine what it would be like to be a helpless little girl with rats chewing on the cast around your neck, with nothing you could do about it.**

Aunt Kit and her brother Bernie stayed up many nights killing huge rats with a baseball bat – trying to keep them away from my mother. At one point, my Uncle Bernie borrowed a BB gun from a friend and, one night, shot and killed rats throughout the night.

Aunt Kit described their first Christmas in Southwest Washington as follows: *"We had no electricity, Mary Ann was still in a cast, and we thought we were going to freeze to death. We did not have any money – NOTHING; but, in the dark still night, we still waited for Santa Claus. On Christmas morning, the Salvation Army brought us a basket. All the toys were used and dirty, but we didn't care. There was also a turkey in the basket, and, on the bottom, there were lots of oranges and apples. In addition, the Harbor Police and firemen from the wharf across the street brought us some food. Dad was still NOT working."*

With the bombing of Pearl Harbor on December 7, 1941, DC changed from a small, sleepy, Southern town to the "Capital of the World" as the U.S. entered World War II. Suddenly, thousands of people were moving into DC, and jobs were available – even to Washington's poorest residents, like my family. My grandmother was able to get steady work at the Greyhound Bus Company. She did minor repairs on the buses and kept them filled with fuel. She loved that job. My grandfather worked intermittently and watched the kids after school.

Slums breed diseases. My grandmother's sister contracted tuberculosis. My mother's sister Bernice visited her in a sanitarium outside of DC. Then, Bernice also contracted tuberculosis, and had to have one of her lungs removed; she lived a long life with just one lung. My grandmother's sister died from her disease – leaving three children that my grandmother cared for in addition to her own five children. Polio was a constant fear of parents during this time because, being in a wheelchair, President Franklin Roosevelt served as a daily reminder of the disease.

My mother and her sisters and brother escaped poverty in different ways. My mother and her sisters, Bernice and Joann, all got married. My Aunt Kit joined the Air Force, Uncle Bernie joined the Marines, and they all went on to have successful, productive families. Aunt Kit became the first single woman to adopt a child in the State of Maryland. My family history consists of many examples of strong, determined, and faithful women who led their families from poverty to success.

By today's standards, my grandparents and parents would be considered to be poor, hardworking people. My dad was a fireman in DC. Both of my parents only had an 8th-grade education. Later, my dad went on to earn his GED and attend college; I remember helping him with his college homework when I was around 10 - 12 years old. My mother was under a huge amount of stress daily. My father was away from home a lot because of his work, going to school, and doing his charity work. My father was also a heavy drinker. My mother and dad married at ages 15 and 17, respectively.

My brother was born when my mother was 16, and I was born 14 months later. My sister was born 10 years after me when our family was in a much better financial situation. My brother had what would now be diagnosed as autism. He was held back a year in first grade, so we were in the same grade. My brother was often bullied at school. I protected him as much as I could. I also helped him with his homework. My parents were extremely happy the day in June 1972 when we both graduated from high school.

My mother and grandmother were self-employed businesswomen who did childcare during the day and cleaned office buildings at night. They were the backbones of their families.

My grandmother encouraged all her grandchildren to have businesses of their own – even if they were side businesses outside of their full-time jobs. She told us, "Nobody gets rich working for someone else." She told us about people she knew who had their own businesses, and how well they were doing. She admired landscapers, plumbers and HVAC repairmen – anyone who worked for themselves. My brother, my sister, and I all had businesses of our own by the time we were adults. In my case, I started my first business when I was a teenager. Also, most of my cousins took her advice and built businesses. She would be SO proud if she were alive today!

My grandmother also told us to own property – the goal being to own your own home as quickly as possible, and then purchase rental houses. My mother and dad owned rental properties from a young age, so I grew up hearing discussions about the tenants, and helping with property maintenance. At an early age, my weekends were spent cleaning, painting, cutting lawns, and doing other repairs with my father. I enjoyed it, and never felt that I was missing out on the other things that kids my age were doing. Watching TV and going to the movies bored me.

COURAGE

"Courage and faith, plus information, defeats fear."
Debbie McGrann

"The most courageous act is still to
think for yourself. Aloud."
Coco Chanel

"Courage is resistance to fear, master of fear
- not absence of fear."
Mark Twain

"With God, you are stronger than your struggles and more fierce than your fears. God provides comfort and strength to those who trust in Him. Be encouraged, keep standing, and know that everything's going to be alright."
Germany Kent

Courage Under Fire

Courage can be taught. In my family I was surrounded by firemen, police officers, and other first responders. These brave people were not fearless. Their training and the information about the situations that they might encounter helped to develop their courage.

Firemen have a strong faith in their fellow firemen. They live together as a family, they sleep at the firehouse, they train at the firehouse, and they share their meals together at the firehouse. When there were emergency situations, they stayed at the firehouse and did not return home until the community was safe again. Members of a fireman's family had to learn to take care of themselves.

I have few memories of my father being with us during holidays. Since our family lived in the DC area, my father worked on holidays to allow the other firemen time off to visit their families outside of the area.

Your life experiences, the lessons that you learn from your mistakes and struggles, develop your courage. Watching how your family and those around you deal with challenges teaches you courage. Also, reading and learning about people who have overcome obstacles and conquered their fears can help you. You learn to be courageous when it is the only option that you have.

When I was first diagnosed with MS, I had faith in my doctors to provide me with the information that I needed to get well. However, I soon learned that I had to have faith in myself to research and find the information that I needed to cure myself.

It took all the courage that I had to refuse the only treatment option that the doctors offered me – drugs. I still remember the hopeless feeling that I had when I left that appointment. Then, I had to battle to hold onto my courage as my symptoms and pain got worse by the day.

Now when I think of courage, I realize that it is something that is within each of us that can be nurtured by faith, information, and learning – ready to appear when we need it. Most of us are stronger than we think. As Coco Chanel stated, "The most courageous act is still to think for yourself. Aloud."

A Childhood in Chaos

I grew up in a small town, Brentwood, Maryland, five miles from the White House. My grandparents lived in the same area, just two blocks from our house. My Aunt Kit, Aunt Joann, Uncle Bernie, and most of my cousins lived within a short drive. We all gathered at my grandparents' house for holidays, birthdays, and Sunday dinners. Our neighbors were like family, and many joined our family for these gatherings. Everyone was welcome at my parents' or grandparents' home.

My Best Friend Kathy's Account During this Period

I was born in Washington, DC. I grew up in the DC suburb of Brentwood, Maryland, one block away from Debbie. Debbie was always the adventurous one. I was the cautious one. I remember one day when my babysitter and I were locked out of my house after school. Fortunately, the small window next to the front porch was unlocked. Instead of having me crawl through it to go inside and unlock the front door, my babysitter recruited Debbie to do it!

Debbie is fiercely loyal to the people she cares about. She looked out for and defended her older brother who had some learning disabilities. She even stood up to a junior high school girl who threatened to beat me up. Thanks to Debbie, the bully left me alone thereafter.

As a child, I was surrounded by hard-working, community-oriented family members, friends, and neighbors. My father was a proud DC fireman. I grew up hearing him and his fellow firemen discussing what they had experienced on a daily basis. As I listened to their stories, their heroic acts became routine for me, and empowered me, as a teenage babysitter, to save a two-year-old child from choking. I also recognized danger when I saw a 3-year-old girl fall into the deep end of a swimming pool and had to dive in to pull her out.

During his 22-year career with the DC Fire Department, my father delivered 57 babies! His delivery kit consisted of a Washington Post newspaper in which to wrap the newborn, and a shoestring to tie the umbilical cord. Later in his career, a nurse provided him with a proper hospital birthing kit.

Firemen risk their lives every day to save others. I watched my brother, a fireman with the airport, on television in January 1981 when an airliner crashed into the Potomac River. I saw him and his fellow firemen rescue passengers from the freezing water. Unfortunately, there were many passengers that they could not reach in time – over which he was deeply stricken with grief.

After my father retired to Florida, he and my mother came to Maryland for a visit. We were at a local restaurant for lunch when the family in the booth behind us suddenly was in a panic because their little boy was choking on a hot dog. The mother shouted for someone to help. My mother told my father, "Go save that boy." My father stood up, and the family passed the boy out of their booth to my father.

As we were passing the boy to my father, our hands on the boy's stomach acted as a Heimlich maneuver, and the hot dog popped out of his mouth; his mother was overjoyed! She thanked my father for his help. My father said that he hadn't done anything. She said, "Yes you did! You stood up!"

If you lived in the DC area in the 1960s and 1970s, you experienced chaos. When I started elementary school in 1960, the U.S. was at the beginning of the Cold War. In school, we had routine "duck and cover" drills to learn how to protect ourselves from nuclear fallout. In our neighborhood, we also had civil defense sirens, and were instructed on how to find the nearest fallout shelter. Some families even built private bomb shelters. Since we were learning in school that DC was the most important city in the world, we knew that we definitely were a prime target for the Russians, and we knew that we were not safe.

In 1957, the Russian's had the successful Sputnik spaceflight. To keep up with the Russians, lawmakers passed the National Defense Education Act, which made American school children important in the Cold War battle. Historian Dee Garrison has stated that students' responses to civil defense drills in schools would later fuel anti-war and antinuclear activism. I remember students having the opinion that since we were all going to die in a nuclear war, we should live for today because we had no future.

At school, we watched all of the American space flights and the splashdowns. These astronauts were the heroes of the 1960s. I was 15 in July 1969 when the United States landed on the moon.

As students, we were also supposed to be physically fit. I remember President Kennedy's Award for physical fitness competitions that we had in elementary school. I looked forward to those game days!

The civil unrest at this time was very frightening to a child. The anger and racial problems of the South were televised for all to see. Martin Luther King had his march on Washington and gave his famous "I Have a Dream" speech. I was in third grade when President Kennedy was assassinated. What a horrible time. The adults all around us were upset and frightened about who had committed this act. Then we watched days of the funeral and were stunned to see his killer murdered on live television. My grandfather died on the same day as the assassination. We had to postpone his funeral because of the Kennedy funeral. We watched as President Johnson took his oath of office in an airplane that was carrying the body of President Kennedy. President Johnson passed the Civil Rights Act and many other changes. In school, we started hearing about a place called Vietnam.

In the United States, the 60s and 70s were a hotbed of political and social upheaval. On February 21, 1965 Malcolm X was also assassinated while addressing his Organization of Afro-American Unity at the Audubon Ballroom in Washington Heights, New York. I was ten at the time.

The Summer of Love was a social phenomenon that occurred during the summer of 1967, when as many as 100,000 people, mostly young people sporting hippie fashions of dress and behavior, converged in San Francisco's neighborhood of Haight-Ashbury. I was not a fan of the hippie movement because of the illegal drug use and the lack of respect for other people that may have disagreed with them.

Tragically, on April 4, 1968, Martin Luther King was murdered, and, that night, Washington burned. As a firefighter, dad was called into duty. He and the other firefighters were attacked with sticks, stones, and crowbars. During the days of rioting that followed, it was reported that the firefighters were helpless; therefore, the National Guard were called in to help. Our neighborhood was so close to the riot that we could smell the smoke and the teargas.

In 1968, after the death of Martin Luther King, Jr in April, there were riots in Washington, DC and across the country. Presidential candidate Robert Kennedy was assassinated on June 6. Of course, these events happened on live television for everyone to watch over and over again.

The Tate murders, in the summer of 1969, emotionally affected the country. Actress Sharon Tate and six persons, which included Sharon's unborn child, were murdered by the Manson Family. They were a group of followers of Charles Manson. They were considered a cult and lived in a desert commune, and often used hallucinogenic drugs.

My teenage years were dominated by racial tension in school that resulted in a large frightening riot in my high school. Police were called in and many students were hurt and arrested. It was even covered by the national media. Students were reacting to forced school busing which precipitated many riots across the country.

Once the draft was reinstated for 18-year-olds, there was an effort to lower the voting age from 21 to 18. There were many chants during the Vietnam War "old enough to fight, old enough to vote." The Twenty-sixth Amendment, lowering the voting age to 18, passed in 1970.

I was a senior in high school during the campaign of the presidential election of 1972. This was the first election in which the voting age was lowered to 18. Because our high school was so close to Washington, DC, we had constant visits and speeches from politicians.

During the presidential campaign of 1972, Arthur Herman Bremer attempted to assassinate U.S. Democratic presidential candidate George Wallace on May 15, 1972, in Laurel, Maryland, which left Wallace permanently paralyzed from the waist down. Our family lived very near to Laurel Maryland; my 18-year-old cousin was in the crowd when the shots rang out. Richard Nixon was elected president in 1972 only to resign in disgrace in August 1974 over the Watergate break-in and impeachment.

My high school adjoined the University of Maryland campus. When the Vietnam protests on the campus of the University of Maryland erupted in riots, the chaos spread to my high school. Our school campus was the site of many anti-war protests. Many college and high school students were arrested. The National Guard was called in to calm the situation, and they occupied the University campus. On May 4, 1970, during an anti-war protest at Kent State University, the National Guard opened fire on the protesters, killing 4 and wounding 9 in Kent, Ohio. Student governments across the country called for school shutdowns and more protests. Again, the University of Maryland was occupied by the National Guard.

The streets of Washington, DC were often crowded with anti-war protests. I remember my father coming home from work after being spit on by anti-war demonstrators. He was attacked while just doing his job to keep the city safe.

The Weatherman Underground group was a left-wing terrorist group. The group was formed in the late 1960s with the intention of advancing communism through violent revolution. The group called on America's youth to create a rear-guard action against the U.S. government that would bring about its downfall.

In October 1969, the Weatherman launched a direct assault on the police by blowing up a statue in Chicago that commemorated the policemen who had died in a riot in 1886. Weatherman members began bombing more targets across the country in 1970. The bombings continued throughout 1971. The Weatherman placed two bombs at the Capitol in Washington, D.C. and both exploded. The Pentagon was also bombed on May 19, 1972. As a D.C. fireman, my father was involved in investigating these bombings.

In my neighborhood, there was chaos in the streets, chaos in the schools, and chaos in families, especially over the Vietnam War. When I was younger, I wanted to be an FBI agent. However, I knew that, as a girl, that was not possible. As I got older, I learned that you should go to law school if you wanted to be an FBI agent. In my family, college for girls was considered a waste of money. My only option would have been the University of Maryland. However, I was not prepared with the higher-level classes required to attend college. When I asked my guidance counselor to arrange for college prep classes for me, she laughed and said, "You are not college material." Unfortunately, I believed her. She would not allow me to take the classes that I needed.

After all of the disruption of my high school years, the continued chaos at the University of Maryland, coupled with a lack of encouragement, made me not want to go to college.

I graduated from High School in June and started working full time in July. Jim and I married in August, and I started to attend college courses at night after working full time during the day. I finished two years of college on a special professional training program before the program was canceled during government cutbacks.

My Career Path

After high school, I started working full-time at NASA as a secretary. I hated the job. After a year in that position, I was able to get a transfer to the library as a research technician. This is where I learned to ask questions of the scientists with whom I was helping with their research projects. I learned where to find the information that they needed for their work. At the time, there was no Internet. Conducting library-type research was similar to being a detective. I loved the job! My boss was very supportive and encouraged me to apply for a special program for college classes. I earned two years of college credits until the program ended.

In my 20s, I played softball on a team at work. I noticed that I was having trouble seeing and developed floaters and flashers in my eyes. I had to stop playing softball. Then, in 1980, I stopped working full time when my daughter, Jennifer, was born. My husband was self-employed, and I helped with his business: I did the entire customer billing for over 4,000 clients. There was no computerized billing at that time. Our son Jimmy was born in 1983.

I started buying investment properties to rent and managed the properties. In 1990, I started a marketing company; and in 1999, I expanded the company.

My Friend Kathy's Account

Although our lives began to take different paths after we graduated from high school, we have remained best friends to this day. Debbie got married and worked as a secretary. I went away to college as a full-time student. I was maid of honor at Debbie and Jim's wedding in 1972.

When I moved back to Maryland, we finally lived close enough to each other to get together whenever we weren't working. We spent a lot of time decorating our houses, watching and discussing soap operas, and drinking vast amounts of hot tea, with a little chocolate on the side. When we became stay-at-home moms, we continued to do those things while our children became friends. We got to share our childhood Ocean City experience with our children when Debbie bought a vacation condo there.

Debbie was always a couple of years ahead of me in life events - getting married, working, having children, buying a house. I always looked to her as a model for how to do all of those things successfully. Our relationship took a new dimension when Debbie and I both started businesses in 1999. Debbie was my first client. To this day, I doubt that I would have had the courage to start the business without Debbie's support and encouragement. I am proud to call myself Debbie's "other sister, Kathy."

My husband worked at night, so he had to sleep during the day. Therefore, I handled most of the school and after-school activities for the kids; and my husband helped as much as he could.

My Daughter Jennifer's Account

My mom was very involved with my brother and me. She was in charge of elementary school events. She came to all of our school activities and sporting events. We would take day trips to Washington, DC, and trips to Disney World.

My mom owned a business and worked from home. She also did paperwork for my dad when he worked for the Washington Post. She was always very busy during the day with working, making dinner, and other activities.

Family Changes

After my father retired, he, my mother, and sister Kathy moved to Florida. I tried to visit them as much as possible. They picked a location based on having friends already there. My father, 42, was very young to retire. His and my mother's "retirement plan" was to build houses and establish a rental property business. They did that, and, over time, came to own 22 rental properties. My father's rental business was based on providing affordable housing for families in the area. He purposely bought and renovated houses for which he could keep the rent low – while still making a small, reasonable profit.

Not satisfied with his house-building business, my father built a restaurant for my mother. My mother then brought the idea of Maryland style cooking of crabs and seafood to Florida by opening MaryAnn's Crab Shack. My mother received rave reviews for her style of cooking, especially for her crab cakes. Financially, it was very successful. In reality, it was too successful! My mother and my father had wanted a small-town restaurant with limited hours, but it turned into a restaurant, a bar, and a private party catering business. It became too much for them to handle, so they sold it to focus on managing their rental properties.

Soon after selling the restaurant, my mother developed breast cancer, and had to have a mastectomy. She left the hospital the day after the surgery because her sister was coming to visit her. She was tough. My father was her caretaker during her recovery period.

In May 2006, my mother suffered a massive aneurism. She was sitting at the kitchen table with my father and neighbors, who had stopped by for a visit. Her condition was grave, and my father had to make the most difficult decision to end her life support after discussing her situation with us kids. As a result of many family discussions, we knew that it was exactly what my mother would have wanted us to do. I told my father that this was going to be the hardest decision that he ever had to do in his life; but it was the right decision to make, because it was what she would have wanted. She died within 30 minutes of being removed from the machines. They had celebrated their 54th wedding anniversary the previous month.

CAREGIVERS

"There are only four kinds of people in the world.
Those who have been caregivers.
Those who are currently caregivers.
Those who will be caregivers, and
those who will need a caregiver."
Rosalyn Carter

"Sometimes asking for help is the most
meaningful example of self-reliance."

from the poem "Sometimes"
by **U.S. Senator Cory Booker**

"Being deeply loved by someone gives you strength, while
loving someone deeply gives you courage."
Lao Tzu, philosopher

CHAPTER TWO

Discovering my Diagnosis

Early Symptoms

My symptoms started slowly, but advanced steadily. At first, my symptoms were so subtle that they did not seem important. When I was a teenager, mother and I made my clothes. We had a system: I constructed the basic dress, and she hemmed it for me. I stood on a low table so she could pin the hem. After a few minutes of standing, I had to sit down. She thought that I had bad circulation in my legs. When I was about 17, I lost a lot of weight. I had never tried to lose weight, so this was alarming! My grandparents had been diagnosed with diabetes, so it was suggested that I get tested, too. As it turned out, I had low sugar (hypoglycemia). So, I was told to eat small meals and snacks throughout the day. My regular activities were not limited by these symptoms.

As I got older, people often commented on how skinny and pale I was. When I was 22, I developed floaters and flashers in my eyes, and was told by "the experts" that there was nothing that could be done about them, and that they were "harmless." But they did interfere with my sight, and I had to stop playing softball for my office team. Also, reading was difficult.

Soon I became pregnant with my first child. I asked my doctor how much weight I should gain during my pregnancy. Because I was so thin, my doctor thought that I should gain 10 pounds. He told me to "gain 10 pounds, and then we would start counting." Jennifer was born in 1980. It was a blessing that I had a normal pregnancy.

Three years later – after my second child was born in 1983, I started having numbness in my feet. Again, taken alone, this was nothing to worry about. But, as I got a little older, I started having dizzy spells and fainting. My doctor said this was caused by low blood pressure (hypotension). His comment, "Be thankful it's not high." However, if you're fainting, and it takes a couple of days to get your blood pressure up to a normal level, it's a problem. I went to see a cardiologist for a second opinion. She told me to drink Gatorade, which would raise my salt and electrolyte levels. This did help.

My Husband's Account

I do recall an incident in which Debbie became so weak, that she fainted, and I had to catch her and lay her on the sofa before she hit the floor.

In the Spring of 2001, I was watching my son play lacrosse. Suddenly, I had double vision and was seeing 2 balls. This was very disturbing to me. I managed to drive home after the game. However, after a couple of days over which my vision did not return to normal, I made an appointment with my eye doctor. After his exam, he told me that I needed to see a neurologist right away. He did not say what he was concerned about. He called the one he knew and got me an appointment for two days later. This seemed serious.

The neurologist scheduled a nerve conduction test, called an electromyogram (EMG). Some conditions that are diagnosed using this test include amyotrophic lateral sclerosis (ALS), Guillain-Barre syndrome, and other serious neurological diseases. In this test, several electrodes are attached to your skin. Then, a shock emitting electrode is placed directly over the nerve, and a recording electrode is placed over the muscles controlled by that nerve. Finally, several quick electrical pulses are given to the nerve.

Since I was driving from a distance about an hour away, I asked the nurse if the test would be painful, and if I should have someone with me to drive me home. She said that no, the nerve conduction test is not painful. She lied; it was VERY painful. Each shock felt like I had stuck my finger into a light socket, and they did over 25 shocks. The technician conducting the test asked me right away if I had someone to drive me home. She was annoyed that the nurse had misled me about the pain and my ability to drive myself home. I drove home, but it was difficult because my nerves and muscles were shaky and weak. This test ruled out ALS as a cause of my double vision.

Next were the blood tests. It was discovered that I had pernicious anemia. I didn't know what "pernicious" meant. On the way home, I stopped at the library to research this condition. I discovered that pernicious means fatal anemia caused by low Vitamin B-12. I noticed that one of the associated diseases was MS; this was the first time that I realized I could have a serious condition. My treatment for pernicious anemia was Vitamin B-12 shots weekly until the numbers were normal, at which time, I could rely on supplements. The neurologist wanted to schedule me for an MRI of the brain.

> **Common sense question:**
> If they could tell my diagnosis from the blood tests, which are easy and not painful, why did they do the painful EMG test first? Was it unnecessary or premature?

Since my next step was going to be an MRI, I decided to switch to a neurologist closer to home. My MRI was September 14, 2001, the same week as the 9/11 attacks.

The first time that I knew what the doctor was looking for was when I was getting ready for my first brain MRI. The nurse asked me what it was like having Multiple Sclerosis (MS). I had not been diagnosed at that time; she read it from my chart. She told me that I "looked good compared to other MS patients." She said that most of the MS patients were brought in by stretcher or wheelchair. The seriousness of my situation began to concern me.

Since I had been undergoing testing for a while, I always requested a copy of my test results. I liked to review the results and do research before I went to the doctors for the follow-up visits. I liked to be prepared with my questions.

I received copies of my brain scan on the same day that I completed the MRI. At home, I held the films up to the light in my kitchen window. I could tell right away something was wrong. The doctor who had reviewed the films had circled a large white spot on my brain and had highlighted it in the comment area. I knew that the white spot was where the problem most likely was located. However, I did not know what the diagnosis would be. Was it MS, a brain tumor, ALS, or something else? I showed the films to my husband. Then we were both worried!

After the MRI, and our unscientific review, we had to wait for the doctor to receive the report from the hospital. We had the film from the scan, but not the accompanying report with the doctor's written interpretation of the film. We had to wait a few days for the doctor to call me to tell me the diagnosis.

The diagnosis was confirmed: Multiple Sclerosis! Then I knew what had been making me so sick for so long. Now, I knew what the enemy was. I was not surprised, but I was confused about what to do. I remember thinking, "Now what do I do? What is the treatment plan? What do I need to do to get better?" Unfortunately, the news was not good. My doctor told me that there was no cure for MS, and that they did not know what caused the disease. The only treatment was experimental drugs that had many side effects. Most patients with MS were known to only get worse over time. My doctor was very matter of fact in explaining my lack of treatment options. There were very few answers for people who suffered from MS. Quite frankly, I felt that my doctor felt lost as well.

On my first visit to my doctor after the diagnosis, he wanted to schedule a spinal tap for me. I had read about spinal taps and the complications associated with having them done. They have to be done in a hospital. One of the side effects of a spinal tap is a headache that can last for several days, and it can be quite severe. I asked him about the side effects. He minimized the chances of side effects. I asked him if he was certain about the results of the MRI, namely, that I had MS. "Yes, you have MS," he replied. "Would the results of this spinal tap change your treatment plan for me?" was my next question. "No" was the answer. "Then, why should I have one?" He replied, "Because I'm really good at it." I knew he was kidding, but I was not in the mood for his humor. I did not think a spinal tap was a good idea; so, I did not have a spinal tap. I felt it was an unnecessary risk to my health, and a waste of my time.

Impact on My Family

My symptoms and pain were worsening by the day, and I was concerned that I was becoming a burden to my family. My daughter was away at college, and my son had taken a job in another state. The main burden of my increasing disability fell on my husband, Jim.

My Husband Jim's Account

I wanted to know what could be done to help Debbie. The diagnosis did not really change Debbie. I was a little fearful of what would be down the road for her, and us. My most intimate fear was that Debbie would be unable to walk. I told her, that despite my fears, I would help in any way I could. Debbie wanted to go on with life as we had in the past, which is very typical of her. Since Debbie was sick, I tried to do as much as I could in terms of household chores.

The one word that my husband used to describe me during this time was Strong!

My Daughter Jennifer's Account

When my mom was diagnosed with MS, I think I tried to ignore it for the most part. I was in college at the time. I was not living at home full-time and pretty involved with my own life, in a self-centered phase. I told myself that MS was not something people died from, which made me feel better. My mom is extremely tough, mentally and physically. It was very rare for her to show that she was having a problem. She never complained to me about anything. I could tell that she was more tired than she used to be and seemed to be in pain sometimes. She continued to work at the same pace. She continued to go to all my brother's sporting events, make dinner every night, etc.

I feared that my mom would continue to get worse and end up in a wheelchair. She is so tough that I didn't realize how bad things were getting. She did not ask for help with anything.

My Best Friend Kathy's Account

The first thing I noticed was that Debbie was unable to eat. We always enjoyed going out to lunch together. I remember taking Debbie to see a lot on which we were thinking about building a house. Since Debbie had already built her own house, I valued her opinion. It was a clear November day in 1992. We visited the lot in the morning, and by lunchtime, we were both starving. We went to Ledo's Pizza, our childhood favorite, for lunch. I quickly devoured my share of the pizza, but Debbie only ate a few bites. She said she would take the rest home to Jim because he would like it. In hindsight, this happened every time we went out to eat; Debbie would order a big meal but wouldn't eat it. Debbie's level of physical activity had also decreased from that of her teenage and young adult years. "Going for a walk" now meant walking around in her back yard or her rose garden. Her pain and double vision (which she didn't talk about) kept her from more strenuous activities.

When I heard her diagnosis, I think I was shocked. It wasn't something I ever expected to hear. I was afraid for her, and I was afraid of losing my best friend. Debbie visited many doctors for both celiac and MS. Their disrespect for Debbie made her more determined to take charge of her own health. Being the cautious, compliant person that, I am, I was afraid that Debbie's decisions not to take the powerful drugs that had possible major side effects was a mistake. I feared she was shortening her life by not complying with her doctors' advice.

Debbie asked me if I would help take care of Jim if she could not. I said I would. Mostly I just listened and asked questions. Debbie had decided how she was going to take charge of her illnesses; there was no need for me to try to convince her otherwise. Debbie asked me to help her address the invitations to her daughter's wedding. (At the time, though, Debbie did not tell me that she asked me to help because her hands hurt. I thought it was because there were a lot of invitations and I had nice handwriting.)

My Cousin Jan's Account

The first time Debbie told me something was wrong was when we were on vacation at Disney World in Orlando in the late 1990s. She said that she was trying to be careful what foods she ate, so she probably would not try anything new in her diet like the alligator sausage that I was excited to try. She said she was being tested for food allergies because it seemed like she was having trouble digesting certain foods. Debbie was worried and downhearted, perhaps lagging behind us. I cannot recall if she had to skip some activities, but I do not recall her being with us all the time. She may have. It would not have been like her to make a big deal of it so I just do not remember, and, at the time, I would never have guessed it was something as serious as MS. I just thought she had a sensitive stomach or food allergies.

The next time I remember was perhaps Mom telling me that Debbie had been diagnosed with MS. I called her at some point and asked her about it. Even then, Debbie did not like to dwell on it, as that is not her way. So, she did not tell me too many details. But Debbie did say that some days she had to stay home and just rest, drink some tea, and perhaps soak in the bathtub to ease the pain. But even then, the pain was still there. I did not get a clear picture of what exactly hurt. I think she said the nerves and the muscles, or just an overall feeling of pain in one or more parts of her body. And, it was not always the same from one day to another. Debbie said I could visit, but she might be resting because she usually had to nap around 2PM. I am sorry to say that I lost motivation and never did get around to visiting. I think I was afraid I would disturb Debbie, and the visit would not really be of any benefit to her. I was glad I had talked to Debbie, but thought a visit might just be tiring for her.

My Sister Kathy's Account

When Debbie became ill, I really wasn't around her much during that time. I was in high school, college, then getting married. There wasn't a lot of time that we spent together. My most immediate reaction to my sister's illness was that the doctors really didn't know and couldn't figure out what was wrong with her. Initially, when she was diagnosed, I thought she was going to die. However, the good news, at least, was that she was able to tell people what she "had." The last time I saw her before she went on her new food plan, she looked horrible. I supported my sister wholeheartedly on her decision not to take medicine. I was there to support her; I really couldn't help in any other way.

When we visited Walt Disney World, I started noticing how sick Debbie was getting. She never had any energy. We had to plan bedtime, so she got enough sleep. When we went into the Park, we would sit and rest more than doing anything else. It was all good to me, but, thinking back, it was a lot of sitting compared to what we do now. When I would go to Debbie's before she was better, I would get up in the mornings and wait for her to get out of bed. A lot of times, it was 10:00 in the morning when she would come down, and then it took a couple hours for her to get moving through the pain and stiffness. We are always joking about whenever she traveled that I had to go with her.

I remember one time I was visiting Maryland, and Debbie was at her worst. I was talking to my husband, Scott, and he asked how she was. I told him she was pretty bad. She looked like an old lady. You could see she was tired; her skin was thin and white, and you could see through to the veins. I told him I wasn't sure what was going to happen with her. She looked bad. She just looked sick.

I had gotten to the point where I was in constant pain. I could not write; when I pressed down on the pen, excruciating pain went up my arm. When I had to use the bathroom or undress, the pressure of pushing my clothes down caused pain so bad that I saw stars and thought I would faint. It was difficult and painful to lift my arms to brush my hair. My husband, Jim had to dry my hair for me because my arms were too weak to hold my hairdryer. Jim also had to button my clothes and tie my shoes. He was a cheerful caregiver, but I was so saddened to add the stress of my care to our lives. With our children grown, this should have been a time for us to relax and enjoy the fruits of our hard work over the years.

My Husband's Account

Debbie was very strong emotionally, so it was hard to notice how she felt.

Disability and serious illness create financial hardships for most families. This was true for my family, too. I was not able to work as much as was required for the business I owned at the time. In addition, we had to draw from our retirement savings. We were grateful that we had been diligent savers for many years.

Divorce is often a side effect of serious illness. In our case, I never had this fear. During my illness and recovery, Jim showed his love for me in the everyday tasks that he did to make my life as normal and as comfortable as possible. He took over all of the household chores that he could while working two jobs. He never complained. During my illness, I tried to shield my family from the consequences of my illness. But my symptoms were getting worse with time, and it was getting harder for me to carry on normal activities.

In July of 2005, our daughter, Jennifer, announced her engagement to her boyfriend, Jason. We were very excited. This not only would be the first marriage on both sides of the family, but it also created the possibility of the first grandchild on both sides of our family! When we started to discuss plans for the wedding, Jennifer told us that she had always dreamed of having her wedding under a tent in our yard. We started to attend many wedding events to get ideas about outdoor weddings. The details were extensive: renting the tent, chairs, tables, glassware, dishes, bar, dance floor, and on and on. We would even have had to rent bathrooms!

We decided to consider indoor options. We all got together to visit different locations. It was a very hot July day. As we were leaving the first location, the heat was starting to make walking difficult for me. When we were all in the car, I told Jennifer that I needed her to have the wedding inside an airconditioned venue. We discussed the heat and what would happen if it was too hot on her wedding day, such that I would not be able to attend her outside wedding. I envisioned the celebration taking place outside in our yard, and me "resting" inside in the air conditioning. In my imagination, I could hear the music and the guests enjoying themselves without me. Jennifer and Jason assured me that they would be fine with having the wedding inside and were very grateful for everything we were doing for the wedding. However, I was very sad that my illness was preventing my daughter from having her perfect dream wedding.

As it turned out, the decision we made that day turned out to be a blessing. My mother died suddenly, six weeks before the wedding that she had been looking forward to attending. We had a celebration of her life at our house the day before Jennifer's wedding. It would have been a logistical nightmare to have had an outdoor wedding in the same yard the next day. Jennifer and Jason had a beautiful wedding inside with air conditioning that we all enjoyed.

If MS is not Fatal, What's Killing Me?

One of the first things the doctor told me after my MS diagnosis was, "Don't worry, it's not fatal." The MS literature says that you do not die from MS, you die with MS. You are still likely to die, probably sooner than you should. However, after suffering from worsening symptoms and declining health, I was beginning to doubt his statement. Also, I began to notice obituaries listing complications from MS as the cause of death. In my case, the outcome appeared bleak. If MS is not fatal, then what's killing me? If MS does not cause pain, then why am I in so much pain? These were important questions to me, but my doctors had no answers to them.

Symptoms Over Time

Starting as a teenager, I had very subtle symptoms: I could not stand for long periods of time, I was very tired, and I had low blood sugar. These symptoms worsened over time. My first serious symptom was diplopia or double vision.

My chronic fatigue grew worse daily until it was in "multi system failure"; I called it "hitting the wall." I felt that my whole body was shutting down, I often got confused, I dropped things, I slurred words to the point that people around me thought I was having a stroke, and I frequently had to lie down to recuperate.

I would "lose" the support of my leg unexpectedly, and I had to hold on to something or someone so that I would not fall. I remember one particular time in my kitchen when I was talking with Jennifer and my leg "disappeared"; luckily, I was able to hold onto the kitchen counter, so I did not fall. I don't think Jennifer realized what had happened. I was really good at hiding my symptoms, especially from my family.

I fell many times due to "foot drop" caused by muscle weakness. I was only bruised by those falls, but they were constant reminders of my MS and my advancing disability. Also, I found it hard to sleep because my muscles would twitch and jump.

I had paresthesia in the form of numbness from my neck down to my toes. I called my physical therapist in the morning after the numbness made it difficult for me to stand when I got out of bed. She advised me to go to the hospital right away. I asked her what they would do for me. She said that they would give me a course of steroids over a couple of days to relieve the numbness. I told her that I would not be going to the hospital because I had decided that I was not going to take steroids. I thought the steroids were a temporary fix, and I also did not want to risk the side effects. I asked her what other option I had. She said, "None. Get a wheelchair and put it in your closet because you are going to need it soon." The numbness lessened over the next couple of days; I still had it, but at least I could walk. I guess I did not need the steroids after all.

Because of the numbness, it was hard for me to feel things. I was cooking one evening and smelled something burning. It was my sweatshirt! It burned through to my skin and left a scar. I didn't even feel it.

I had painful burning sensations in random places on my body. I had cognitive dysfunction on a daily basis. Because of this mental impairment, I made some bad business decisions.

By 2005, I had terrible pain in my ears. The pain radiated to my upper neck. It was worse when I laid down, which made sleeping difficult and painful. I had tinnitus in both ears, which caused my hearing to be distorted when I was in a group setting. Because of my hearing problems, I did not want to be around people. It was embarrassing to have to keep asking them to repeat themselves or to misunderstand what they said. I was becoming antisocial, and I did not like that feeling.

I went to an ear, nose and throat doctor for testing. I explained my situation and told him that, "I hope I have a brain tumor." He reviewed my latest MRI report and told me, "I'm sorry, you don't have a brain tumor." We both laughed at how ridiculous that sounded. He told me that he knew why I was hoping for the brain tumor: if I had a brain tumor, the solution would be to cut the tumor out, and the pain would be relieved. However, if the pain was a symptom of MS, there was no solution, and the pain would probably get worse. He told me that he had an uncle with MS, so he understood my reasoning. He then gave me some good advice, saying that most diseases are managed, not cured.

Around this time, my brother, around 55 or younger, told me that he had been diagnosed with osteoporosis. I thought that, if he had osteoporosis, there was a good chance that I had it, too. He and I had most of the same risk factors for osteoporosis: tall, thin, fair, blue eyes, and family members with the disease. Neither one of us had ever smoked.

I started to wonder why my doctor had not recommended this test for me since I was over 50. I scheduled a bone density test for myself. When my doctor's office received the results from the bone density test, a staff member called me. She was very annoyed. She wanted to know, "Who ordered this test?" I told her that I had ordered this test for myself. She told me, "That's not the way it should be done." I thought, "Oh, well!" Apparently, if it was going to get done, it was up to me to do it. I made an appointment to meet with the doctor.

Before my appointment, I received a letter from the doctor. She mentioned that my test did show significant bone loss in both my spine and hip, which meant that I had osteoporosis in both regions. She mentioned that she had not seen me in four years. I had last visited her after I was diagnosed with MS. I told her about the pain I was having in my back and hips. Knowing my family history and my other risk factors, I think she was realizing that she should have suggested that I have a bone density test much earlier, and because of that delay, I now had severe osteoporosis with little hope of reversing the damage. I'm sure that is why I received her letter.

At my appointment with her, she emphasized how bad my bones were. It was raining on the day of my appointment, and she pointed out the window at the bad weather and told me to go home and not go out in the bad weather. She was concerned about the combination of bad balance from my MS, and my fragile bones. She was afraid that I would fall and break a bone. She prescribed Fosamax for me.

I had a terrible reaction to Fosamax after taking the first dose. It felt like burning acid was going through my bones. I had severe and painful diarrhea with bloody stools. I had never had such a horrible reaction to anything in my life. I called the doctor to let her know about my reaction, and to see if there was anything else, I could do. She said she was on vacation and would get back to me.

A few days later, I received another letter from her. She acknowledged that my bone loss was significant from the previous test. She recommended that I speak to someone about it. She stated, "I am not sure what to do." She said that, because of my serious side effects, I could not continue taking Fosamax. I felt like she was firing me as a patient and documenting the reasons for legal cover.

I thought that I must be a very difficult case since she was telling me that she did not know what to do to help me. I felt alone in the battle for my health. At that point, I was in horrible pain every day and desperate for answers. I was disappointed that she had no further suggestions for me. I thought, "What do I do now to help myself get better?" Once again, I concluded that my healing had to be up to me.

TIME

"Your greatest resource is your time."
Brian Tracy

"Time is more valuable than money. You can get more money, but you cannot get more time."
Jim Rohn

"Don't wait for things to get easier, simpler, or better. Life will always be complicated. Learn to be happy right now. Otherwise you'll run out of time."
Lessons Learned in Life, Inc.

TIME?

Time. How much did I have left? As my symptoms worsened, I started to be very conscious of every decision about how I spent my time. One reason that I avoided taking drugs was the amount of time it would steal from my life. One of the most common side effects was flu-like symptoms for 2-3 days after the monthly shot of the MS drugs. That added up to a total of 36 additional sick days a year; I was not willing to give up more time to be sick.

I spoke with my friend Kathy about the best use of my time. I asked her to encourage me to host a family event at least once a month. I did not want my illness to steal my precious time with family and friends. I was very purposeful in hosting the holiday dinners for my extended family. I hosted birthday dinners for my children and other family members. I also hosted Sunday dinners, and visited my family in Florida. I wanted to create lasting memories for my husband and children.

I hosted a 75th birthday party for my father. At the party was a dear family friend, Alice, with whom we had been very close for many years. When she left the party, my sister and I walked her to her car to spend more time with her. After we hugged her goodbye, we knew that it might be the last time that we would see her, and, unfortunately, it was. I know that those last few minutes were as meaningful to her as it was to us. At the party, I wondered if anyone thought it would be the last time that they would see me.

I learned a lesson that day: minutes count and spend time with your loved ones every minute you can. Sometimes when I did something special or even ordinary family events, I wondered if it would be the last time that I was going to be healthy enough to participate. After making Christmas dinner in 2007, I was so exhausted that I could not eat my food. I went upstairs to lie down and rest for a few minutes. I could hear the sounds of joy from downstairs, and I was saddened to think that I likely would be spending the rest of my holiday dinners away from everyone.

As time went on, I decided to spend less time watching television, and more time reading and learning. After New Year's Day 2008, I started to spend a lot of time researching my illness and possible treatments. This was time well spent because it saved my life!

Your time becomes more precious when you think you are running out of it. Time is a priceless commodity, especially when you actually are running out of it. When you are out of time, you are out of everything. Spend it wisely.

My Pain Became My Information

As I started to think of myself as a medical detective, I began to look at my pain in a different way. I came to realize that my pain was information and evidence.

I realized that I needed to examine that information to discover the source of my pain. That was my goal, to determine:

- What is causing all my pain? and
- What is the source of my pain?

Pain can be a great motivator. My motivation was to find the source of my pain before it got unbearable. I had read that suicide rates were very high in MS patients because of the pain, disability, and lack of hope. Depression is another side effect of chronic pain. I protected myself from depression by purposely filling myself with positive thoughts.

Other MS patients had told me how marijuana had helped them with their pain. Since I was a resident of Maryland and suffering from chronic pain, I would have been able to get medical cannabis. Once again, I thought that the side effects of taking this drug were not worth the risk. I was happy for the other patients who had found something to help them manage their pain. However, I was concerned that the marijuana was just masking their pain. I wanted to find the source of my pain. To solve this part of the puzzle, I knew that I had to gather the facts:

Question: *What type of pain did I have? Muscle pain? Bone pain?*
Answer: I had both types of pain.

Question: *Where was the pain? In my back? In my hips? All over?*
Answer: My pain was all over. It seemed to start in my back and hips.

Question: *When was the pain the worse? In the morning? At night?*
Answer: My pain was moderate in the morning. I felt better after a warm shower. The pain worsened as the day wore on. My pain caused me to wake up many times during the night.

Question: *Was it getting worse over time?*
Answer: The pain was getting worse each day.

Question: *Was there anything that made the pain better? A hot shower? An ice bath?*
Answer: I found that a warm shower in the morning helped. Also, later in the day, I put my feet in cold water, which seemed to help.

Question: *How bad was the pain?*
Answer: At first the pain was manageable. But the fact that the pain was getting worse worried me.

Question: *Could I sleep through the night?*
Answer: I could not sleep through the night.

Question: *Could I stand for more than 15 minutes?*
Answer: No, I could not stand for more than 15 minutes. The longer I stood, the worse the pain got.

Question: *How long could I work before I had to lie down?*
Answer: As time went on, my workday became shorter; I could work for about four hours before I had to "rest."

Question: *Was the pain worse in the heat? In the cold?*
Answer: Heat made my pain much worse. Heat also made my muscles very weak. When my muscles became weak, it was harder to walk, and tripping became a problem. Cold was better for me.

Question: *Why was the pain getting worse?*
Answer: I did not know "why" my pain was getting worse, but I was determined to find out.

There is a vicious cycle to pain: Pain causes stress, and stress makes pain worse. By looking at my pain as information, I took much of the stress and emotion out of it. This allowed me to think much more clearly about possible solutions. As I analyzed and researched my pain, I came closer to my cure.

DEBBIE MCGRANN

PERSISTENCE

"If you are going through hell, keep going."
Winston S. Churchill

"Never, never, never give in!"
Winston S. Churchill

"The three great essentials to achieve anything worthwhile are, first, hard work; second, stick-to-itiveness; third, common sense."
Thomas Edison

CHAPTER THREE

I Learned to Always be Persistent

Persistence

I realized that my best, and some might have suggested, my worst trait was being persistent because I never gave up no matter how bad my situation appeared. After I was diagnosed with MS, surrendering to my illness and the constant pain was never an option for me because I was in a battle for my life. It was important for me to be determined regardless of the situation in which I found myself. I always remembered the saying "This, too, shall pass."

Marching Onward

My symptoms became much worse. I had double vision in both eyes. My muscles became very weak, which made walking very difficult. I lost hearing in both ears, and I was in constant pain. The pain was excruciating and made simple daily tasks like getting dressed very difficult. Also, I felt like I was running out of time. I could tell that my husband, Jim, and my children were very worried about my future. Most people that I told about my condition were very saddened and expressed surprise and sympathy.

I reasoned that drugs were the wrong treatment for me. I thought that the side effects of the drugs that my doctors were willing to prescribe would make me worse. Instead, I instinctively knew that I had to find the source of my pain. As a result, I decided to rely on my own research and faith to solve my problem and to find a solution to my medical mystery. As a first step for this phase of my journey, I started thinking about my family medical history. I had seen my grandmother and my mother steadily decline before they died, and I did not want that to happen to me. I was determined to find out how to stop my own decline.

I asked God for the strength to handle what was coming my way. In addition, I often gave myself pep talks – telling myself that I could handle anything. I was certain that my doctors and other health practitioners were missing something. I realized that I should trust my ability to handle problems, and also not to rely on most of the information that others gave me. In effect, I decided to "trust but verify." More importantly, I decided to keep researching until I found the answers that I needed to heal my body.

DEBBIE MCGRANN

CURIOSITY

"I have no special talent. I am only passionately curious."
Albert Einstein

"The important thing is not to stop questioning. Curiosity has its own reason for existing."
Albert Einstein

"Curiosity is more important than knowledge."
Albert Einstein

"Curiosity is the best remedy for fear."
Unknown

CHAPTER FOUR

I Was Chosen: "Why me?" "Why not me?"

I never asked, "Why me?" I had a feeling that I had been chosen to have MS for a reason, though, at first, I was not sure what the reason was. However, I came to know that I had been chosen to have MS because I was the type of person who would search until I found the answers that I needed to survive this ordeal, and that I would be the person who would witness to others. I was humbled by the fact that such an important mission was entrusted to me. By having MS and recovering, I would be able to inform not only my family members and their future generations about Celiac Disease and its impact on their health, but also the same for countless others around the globe.

When I was first diagnosed with Multiple Sclerosis and started the search for answers and my cure, I realized that the strength of my curiosity would determine the success of my mission.

As I started to recover from MS and share my story with others, my true purpose in life was clearly revealed: My mission in life was my duty and responsibility to share my story so that others could benefit from my discoveries, and thereby enjoy healthier, happier lives. It was time to get started!

Why?

I was born with a strong sense of curiosity. As a child, I was always asking questions. I wanted to know how everything worked. "Why?" was my favorite word! When I started school, I soon learned that some teachers did not like to be asked "Why?"

For example, I remember when I was in second or third grade and asked the teacher, I'm sure repeatedly, "Why is the ocean salty?" At the time, we were discussing the ocean, but she did not answer my very relevant question. Of course, I kept asking. She told me to "sit down and shut up!" I was very surprised and upset. After school, I went to my grandparents' house. My grandfather could tell that I was upset. He asked me what my problem was. I told him what my teacher had said, and I told him that she was mad at me.

He told me to never stop asking questions. He said that some people will get mad when people ask questions because they don't know the answer. Instead of taking time to find the answer to the question, they get mad. He also reminded me that it was my responsibility to find the answers, too. Also, a teacher has lots of children asking her questions all day. (This was before the Internet and searching for answers often took a considerable amount of time.) He brought out his encyclopedia and we looked up the information we needed to answer my question. He also taught me that it was not necessary to know all the answers in life, but it was necessary to know how to find the answers when they were needed.

My best friend Kathy remembers a time when my curiosity caused me a little trouble:

"Debbie was always full of curiosity – as in 'I wonder what would happen if I ...' A memorable consequence of Debbie's curiosity occurred when she removed the head of a water fountain in our elementary school (Thomas Stone Elementary), thereby flooding the school. The image of water rushing down the stairs from the second to the first floor of the school is still vivid in my memory."

I remember that day, too. The teacher was very upset.

As I got older, the skill of knowing how to find the answers to my own questions grew into a lifetime of self-education and learning. I used these skills when I worked at NASA helping scientists with their research projects (still no Internet!). This skill also saved my life when I had to become a medical detective to cure my "incurable MS."

The Discovery Process

They said that they did not know the cause of MS, and that there was not a cure for MS. Of course, at first, I felt discouraged, lost, and hopeless. However, deep within my heart, I strongly believed that they were missing something. My instincts told me that there was more to learn.

Also, I was discovering the pattern of doctors being arrogant, and, many times, outright wrong! They told me what they thought I should do about my illness. When I questioned them or told them that I would not do what they wanted me to do, they got very agitated.

Oftentimes, doctors don't like to be questioned. One doctor even told me to leave! Unfortunately, I discovered that I was not the only patient who was experiencing this treatment. Friends with other illnesses were having the same reactions from their doctors.

Searching for Answers

After my diagnosis in 2001, I was discouraged with my lack of treatment options. It appeared that if I declined the drug treatment, there would be nothing left for me to do. It seemed as though the doctors were just going to stand back and watch as my disability increased. Then, I was told about a special complementary medicine program at a local hospital for Multiple Sclerosis patients – the University of Maryland Hospital. I had my first appointment in August of 2002, almost a year after my initial diagnosis.

This program was different. The doctors acted more like consultants and were more curious than the doctors I had been seeing. Also, they spent more time with me, and were not pushing the drug therapy option. They scheduled me for an update on all of my blood tests. For example, I knew that I had a Vitamin B-12 deficiency, so I continued to take Vitamin B-12 supplements. When the results of my blood tests came back, my vitamin D level was extremely low. The pharmacist told me that it was the lowest level he had ever seen. I read a book on vitamin D deficiency, which indicated that it could be the cause of my bone pain. I immediately started taking Vitamin D supplements, but I did not notice any reduction in the pain in my bones.

They also tested me for Lyme disease, which was negative. The University of Maryland program was going through some sort of reorganization, and the doctors changed frequently. This meant that I had to start over with a new doctor at each visit. They renamed the center to University of Maryland Integrative Medicine, LLC.

I continued to go to this center because I thought it was my best hope for getting the information that I needed for my recovery. By December 2007, my most recent doctor was leaving, and I wanted to have an appointment with her before she left. When I arrived for my appointment, I was startled by her comment: "Debbie, I'm concerned about you. You are getting really bad really fast." I told her that I was concerned about me, too. I then asked her, "What should I do?" Her response was "I don't know."

Oh no, another dead-end, and I was at a center that specialized in Multiple Sclerosis. What do I do now? Who can help me? I asked her if she thought I had a malabsorption disorder. Her reply: "I don't know." I asked her about the possibility of malabsorption as an explanation – thinking about my low vitamin levels for Vitamin B-12 and Vitamin D, as well as low sugar levels, and low body weight. These levels had remained low even after increasing my vitamin dosages and trying to gain weight. She suggested that I go to an endocrinologist, and also to a personal trainer to build strength. I wished her well on her move back to her home state of Oregon.

On the way home, I stopped by a gym to consult with a personal trainer that I knew. I told him that I needed to build strength because of my osteoporosis and MS. I also told him that I was in a lot of pain. He replied, "If you think you are in pain now, wait until I'm done with you." This did not seem like a good plan for me because he did not know the source of my pain. It seemed like a bad idea to start a training program without first finding out why I was in so much pain. Another dead-end! Was there anyone who knew what to do to help me? I was beginning to doubt it.

New Year's Eve 2007, after my last visit at the University of Maryland Integrative Medicine Center, I gave up on doctors helping me with my recovery. I decided that if I was going to get better and not die, I had to find the answers myself. I decided, *"If it's going to be, it's up to me!"* I felt empowered and confident that I could solve this problem. I was excited to get started on my new mission to save my life! I told my husband, "buckle up, its going to be a wild ride!" I think he was encouraged by my determination and renewed mental strength.

I decided to spend less time watching television, and more time reading and learning. After New Year's Day 2008, I started to spend a lot of time researching my illness and possible treatments. This was time well spent because it saved my life!

My search for answers began the next day, New Year's Day 2008. Let the battle begin!

DEBBIE MCGRANN

FEARLESS

"I do not fear that my words will offend someone because I have confidence that my words will inspire someone."
Debbie McGrann

"Once you make a decision, the universe conspires to make it happen."
Ralph Waldo Emerson

"Nobody's life is ever all balanced. It's a conscious decision to choose your priorities every day."
Elisabeth Hasselbeck

"The time to take counsel of your fears is before you make an important battle decision. That's the time to listen to every fear you can imagine! When you have collected all the facts and fears and made your decision, turn off all your fears and go ahead!"
General George S. Patten

CHAPTER FIVE

Becoming Fearless

New Year's Day 2008

My decision on New Year's Day 2008 was to take charge of my situation. I decided to consider doctors as consultants and not bosses. My judgment of doctors changed because I then realized that their reactions were caused simply by a lack of knowledge about treatments other than drugs for MS. I had had two doctors tell me that they didn't know what to do. If I was going to live, I had to figure it out on my own. My motto had been, *"If it's going to be, it's up to me!"*

On New Year's Day 2008, I announced to my family that my resolution for the New Year was to cure my MS. I was surprised by the negative reactions of some of my family. My father-in-law asked me, "Who do you think you are? You are not a doctor. What makes you think you can cure Multiple Sclerosis?" I was surprised at his hostile tone, but I told myself that this was what I was going to encounter from a lot of people, so I had better have a good answer for him. My response was, "I know I am not a doctor. I asked my doctor if he knew what causes MS and he said no. I asked my doctor if he knew what the cure for MS was and he said no. So, I know as much about my MS as he does. Plus, I have more time to research my MS than he does."

After I made the decision to cure my MS on my own, I started to think of myself as a medical detective. I was going to search everywhere for the answers to my health issue. I was either going to get better or die trying! My receptive brain power was now fully engaged. When the student is ready, the teacher comes.

The first week of January 2008, my business associate, Rich, came to my home office to pick up some documents. He knew that I had MS, and he had previously asked me for advice for his sister-in-law, Nancy, who had been diagnosed after me. Before he left, I asked him how Nancy was doing. His answer jolted me to the core! "She's cured." "She's cured? Doctors usually do not use the words cured and MS in the same sentence," I responded. He replied, "I agree, but that's what her doctor told her." "That is wonderful news. Do you know what cured her?" I asked. "They changed her diet – something about wheat," he said.

He gave me her phone number so I could contact her. I called her later that same day and explained what Rich had told me about her cure. She told me that it was all about her diet, but she did not go into detail. She gave me the contact information of her doctor. Unfortunately, I had asked her the wrong question. Instead of asking for her doctor's contact information, I should have asked her more about her diet. Thus, I missed an opportunity because I did not know how important her diet was to her cure, and she was in a hurry to get off the phone to get her children from school. But the conversation was filed away in my brain for later use.

In April of 2008, I went to my local library on one of my many visits to research MS. There was a display of books about autism in the lobby. April was Autism Awareness Month. I checked out a book by Jenny McCarthy, *Louder Than Words*. I stayed up late into the night reading it.

Louder Than Words is a book about Jenny McCarthy's fight to find a cure for her son's autism. Her answers came from accidental information that she discovered from other mothers. She received little help from the medical community and was often scorned for her belief that a diet could help her son recover from autism. However, the mothers that she met in her search for treatment for her son empowered her. I could relate to her experiences with her search for answers, and I found strength in her fight for her son's cure.

According to the website, generationrescue.org, her book and nationwide speaking tour sparked a movement of mother warriors empowered to take control of their families' health and well-being.

Wow! Here was a national celebrity having trouble with her son's doctors not offering any hope for her son's autism and treating her with disrespect. I was having the same trouble with the medical community that she and her family were having. I felt like I had met a kindred spirit.

There is no drug treatment for autism. Unlike my struggle to decide whether to take MS drugs, children with autism do not have that option. Their families had to seek answers in other treatments from the get-go. A gluten-free diet was their only option for recovery for their children. After reading this book, I began to think about diet in a different way. Could diet cause and cure diseases? Could diet cause and cure MS? Was this a clue for me?

Mother's Day 2008 - A Critical, Impactful Decision

My daughter Jennifer invited us to visit North Carolina and spend Mother's Day with her and her husband, Jason. Since my mother had died the week of Mother's Day 2006, I was glad to make the trip.

On Saturday, Jennifer treated me to tea at a local hotel, where we had a chance to discuss my research about the horrible bone pain I was experiencing. I had some new information that I wanted to share with her and get her opinion. Jennifer, my sister Kathy, and my friend Kathy were my sounding board for all the information I was discovering in my quest to cure my MS. The more we talked, the more we realized that we could be on to something valuable.

On the way home, we stopped at a bookstore to see if we could find anything useful. The focus of our search was a word new to both of us: GLUTEN. I had been seeing this word repeatedly in the research that I was doing. Although this word was new to us, the bookstore had several books on the subject. Jennifer took a book and I took another book. As we scanned the list of symptoms, we realized that we might be on to something new and important. The list of symptoms in both books matched my symptoms! Jennifer told me that I was the poster child for gluten intolerance – also known as Celiac Disease.

Gluten-free for Dummies was my Mother's Day gift to me and my family. I spent the rest of the day reading it and became very excited about all the new information I was discovering! For the first time since I had been diagnosed, I felt hopeful. After dinner, I announced that I was going to be gluten-free – starting in the morning. None of us knew exactly what this meant and what the impact would be. I finally had a plan of action to fight this illness (whatever it was)!

Mother's Day morning is usually a time for donuts. Since this was my first day being gluten-free, I passed on the donuts and, instead, had a cup of tea and a banana. On the drive home, I continued to read, *Gluten-free for Dummies*, and studied the diet guidelines. For lunch, my husband and I stopped at McDonald's. The book listed McDonald French fries as being gluten-free, so I had French fries and sweet tea for lunch. For dinner, I had McDonald French fries, tea, and a banana. When we arrived home, I was still hungry, so I made scrambled eggs.

I was so excited by this diet plan that I could hardly sleep. In summary, all I ate that first day was tea, bananas, McDonald French fries, and scrambled eggs. My KISS diet plan: Keep It Simple Stupid! So far, so good! The next day, I awakened feeling more refreshed than usual. Jennifer called and asked how I was feeling. I told her that I thought I was better. "It could be psychological" was her opinion. "I'll take that!" was my reply. I was happy for any positive reaction from my body.

My Best Friend Kathy's Account

Once Debbie adopted a gluten-free diet, she could eat a full meal again. She ate like a person who had been starving – which she was. She began to gain weight once her food no longer made her sick. I suppose I was skeptical but hopeful. There wasn't as much information connecting inflammation and chronic illnesses at that time as there is now. Instead of simply masking the symptoms of MS with drugs, Debbie addressed her Celiac Disease, which caused her MS.

How could my doctors not have told me about this diet? Did they not know? Although I had been treated by more than 13 doctors for over 25 years, not one of them had suggested this simple treatment to me.

Multiple Sclerosis, lupus, Crohn's disease, fibromyalgia, osteoporosis, arthritis, diabetes, migraines, chronic fatigue, and more, are all autoimmune conditions that may be helped or cured with the same treatment that I had found to be successful. Today, many patients are getting better on a gluten-free diet. Has your doctor suggested this simple treatment for you, or are they only pushing drugs? Many have undiagnosed Celiac Disease, which is causing one or more other autoimmune disorders.

My doctor told me that MS was not fatal, although I felt like I was dying. Then I knew that I was dying, starving to death, and facing death. Left untreated, Celiac Disease can be fatal. Is this what's killing you? I would recommend that you go on a gluten- free diet to see for yourself if you get better. Unlike drugs, a gluten-free diet has no dangerous side effects. Are you ready to be well?

DEBBIE MCGRANN

FAITH

"Truly I tell you, if you have faith as small as a mustard seed, you can say to this mountain, 'Move from here to there,' and it will move. Nothing will be impossible for you."
Matthew 17:20

"I want to be a woman who overcomes obstacles by tackling them in faith, instead of tiptoeing around them in fear."
Renee Swope

"Believe in yourself! Have faith in your abilities! Without a humble but reasonable confidence in your own powers, you cannot be successful or happy."
Norman Vincent Peale

CHAPTER SIX

A Measure of Faith

Faith

We all are given some faith. Even if your faith is as small as a mustard seed, you can build on that and find strength and hope. I strengthened my faith in myself. I started to be very intentional about focusing and building on my faith.

I planted seeds of faith every day in every way that I could. I went to the store and bought mustard seeds to put in my pocket. During the day, if my pain was really bad, I reached into my pocket and felt the mustard seeds as a reminder that I could conquer this situation.

I fed my faith daily. I read the Bible, focusing on passages of encouragement. I took some of the quotes that are in this book and wrote them on note cards. Every day, I reviewed the cards in the morning and at night. I even made an extra set to keep in my car. Also, I read motivational books about people who had overcome various obstacles in their lives, including fighting illnesses. I read books about business leaders and their paths to success. I gave myself pep talks to tamp down my doubts, and I talked with trusted family members and friends about my diagnosis. I was then ready to make my miracle happen!

Maintaining a Positive Mental State

Whenever you are faced with a debilitating disease, you must maintain a positive attitude while you go through the healing process. Therefore, I knew I that I had to keep myself motivated and focused. To do this, I started reading. Daily, I read several verses of the Bible. My favorite verses were:

"I can do all things through Christ who strengthens me."
Philippians 4:13 (KJV)

"If ye have faith as a grain of mustard seed, ye shall say unto this mountain, remove hence to yonder place; and it shall remove; and nothing shall be impossible unto you…"
Matthew 17:20 (KJV)

I also read motivational books by Joel Osteen, who really spoke to my heart, and helped me to maintain a positive perspective; I often taped his TV programs. If one of his messages was reassuring, I listened to it multiple times. I looked up his cited Biblical messages for added comfort and inspiration. Also, I listened to positive business leaders in the car on the way to and from my office.

In addition, I enjoyed reading great books like *The Power of Positive Thinking,* by Norman Vincent Peale, and *Think and Grow Rich* by Napoleon Hill. I also read two books by Robert H. Schuller: *Tough Times Don't Last, But Tough People Do!* and *If It's Going to Be,*

It's Up to Me: The Eight Proven Principles. Furthermore, I read a variety of books on business leaders who had overcome hardships to become successful (Most of them had had hardships and failures early in their lives). Great leaders like Henry Ford and Milton Hershey had to overcome many obstacles early in their childhoods before they reached their pinnacles of success.

It is critical that you learn to give yourself pep talks. When I was having a really bad day, I called my best friend Kathy, who joked that she would get her pom poms ready. The thought of her with pom poms always lifted my spirits.

I told myself that I could live with the pain and disability that I already had, but that I needed to find a way to keep it from getting worse. I told myself that it could be worse, so I focused on what I could still do. When I fell or stumbled (which was happening more frequently), I used humor to get through the moment. I found my confusion with words to be the most embarrassing and hardest with which to deal. When it happened, I felt stupid, and knew that people did not realize that the confusion was part of a disease, since I didn't outwardly look sick. Some thought I was having a stroke or was drunk; it was confusing to them, too.

I was not able to exercise much because of the fear of falling due to my balance problems. However, I did go to physical therapy sessions, and I tried to keep up a work schedule; but, because of my extreme fatigue, my workdays got shorter and shorter. Also, because of my speech and hearing problems, meeting with people was becoming more difficult.

From 2001 to 2011, my husband Jim and I attended Penn State home football games on Saturdays. Although the travel to and from the games was painful, I enjoyed being around so many people.

(They were strangers, so if I walked funny, I didn't care.) As my symptoms worsened, the pain in my ears was intensified by the noise in the stadium. Luckily, I could leave my seat and watch the game from another less-loud area. I enjoyed being around all the music and festivities of the game. I also enjoyed being around healthy and excited young people. Jim loved going to the games, and I enjoyed seeing him having such a good time and not having to help me! It took away a lot of stress for the day.

I told everyone that I had MS – even strangers. I thought that perhaps I could encourage them since everyone tended to say, "but you look so good." Of course, I realized that pain is not always visible. Also, since I was pretty sure that my doctors were missing something, maybe a stranger would have some insight that would help me. I also told everyone with whom I worked about my stumbling and balance issues because I wanted them to know what was wrong.

I still had a business to run. I worked from home but had to see clients as much as possible in order to earn money for the business. I had an assistant who came two to three days a week. As I got sicker, my workday became shorter. I could not get up and going before 10am, and I had to "rest" in the middle of the day. My assistant left at 3 pm each day. Also, I had to rest a little more before starting dinner, which we usually ate at 6 pm. Sometimes, I was too tired to eat, and it was becoming hard to swallow. My husband, Jim did all of the cleanup. I was in bed by 8 pm, and I did my reading and studying from 8 to 9 pm.

Luckily, a few doctors had told me that they did not know what to do for me. That's when I finally, fully realized that I had to take control of my situation or I would die! I started by strengthening my confidence that, in real life, I could find the answers that I needed.

I started at the public library by reading every book that I could find on MS and other related illnesses. I thought about it all of the time – wondering what my doctors had been missing, and what else could be wrong. In 2006 my mother died. As I looked through pictures for her memorial service, I noticed how much weight she had lost before she died. My grandmother had experienced the same thing – "wasting away." The same thing was happening to me: I could not gain weight or keep the weight that I previously or recently had. Therefore, I started searching for "wasting disease" in medical information sources. Also, I asked my sister about wasting disease in animals.

My Sister Kathy's Comments

I went to the doctors to get a physical because of Debbie's illness. The day that I came out of the doctor's office and called her to tell her that the doctor had said I had nothing wrong with me, but he said that I would feel better if I lost 5 pounds. I told him no, won't do that, all the women in our family die at 90 pounds from losing weight in their later years. That was when we both realized that there was something going on in our family. Debbie searched wasting diseases and narrowed it down to gluten intolerance. It made sense.

In 2008, I became laser focused about finding answers because I had to: I was getting really bad. I still asked questions of my doctors; however, I now considered them consultants, and not people with all of the answers. I wrote down everything they told me, I asked follow-up questions, and I even asked them to spell terms with which I was not familiar. They found this annoying, but I did not care what they thought because my life depended on my finding answers fast.

I think that, when I was initially diagnosed with MS, the doctors put me in "the MS box." This provided a context such that they had stopped looking for other solutions because they thought that MS was the singular, final answer; they had no awareness about Celiac Disease and how it was related to MS. They had become intellectually lazy. They received all of their information about MS and MS treatments from the pharmaceutical companies, and they had stopped being curious.

GRIEF

"Accept what is. Let go of what was.
And have faith in what will be."
Zig Ziegler

"Grief is in two parts. The first is loss.
The second is the remaking of life."
Anne Roiphe

"Nobody can bring you peace but yourself."
Ralph Waldo Emerson

Reaction to Recovery

Within days of starting my gluten-free diet treatment, I was obviously better. I called my business partner, Marsha, about a project we were working on together. She asked how I was feeling. I told her that I was having a great day, and I told her about my new treatment. She said that she could tell something was different because my voice was much stronger; I heard similar comments from other people with whom I talked that week – just a few days after starting my new diet!

I also called Nancy to tell her how much better I was feeling, and to thank her for her help. I thought it was important for her to know that she had given me the hint that food could be my cure just like how she had been cured. I commented to her that my daughter Jennifer said I should write a book about my recovery. She responded, "There already is a book – *The MS Recovery Diet*. I was so surprised! I thanked her for her help, and immediately went to Barnes & Noble to see if I could buy or order the book; they had it on the shelf! I spent the rest of the day and into the night reading and rereading the book!

I was amazed at the information I was reading. This book described case studies of patients with MS who recovered from diet alone, just like me. Some patients were bedridden but recovered when they adopted a gluten-free diet! Why was I not told about this book? Did my doctors not know this information?

My neighbor, Janet, had MS, too. I learned of her diagnosis when my daughter, Jennifer, participated in an MS walk to raise money. Janet thanked her for walking for her, too. The day after I read the book, I went to Janet's house to tell her about the information.

She knew nothing about the book or the diet. I found it incredible that eating the right food could cure MS, but that no one was talking about it.

I was surprised at how I reacted to this revelation. In part, I was angry because my doctors had discussed drugs as the only treatment for MS. In addition, I was angry that the pharmaceutical industry incentivized doctors to prescribe their drugs, but never mentioned that eating the proper foods could cure MS. I was also angry because the various media only pushed drugs, too! Every "new" treatment for MS was a dangerous drug – with never a mention about the cheaper, safer, and more effective dietary treatment. In addition, I was angry at the American culture of pill-popping vs. changing diet and lifestyles. It seemed that doctors assumed that their patients would not follow a dietary treatment (if they ever knew about such a treatment), and, instead, prescribed drugs without giving them the information that they needed to make intelligent decisions for themselves.

When my grandmother was diagnosed with diabetes in the 70s, she was given a diet plan to follow, which she did religiously. Today, she likely would immediately be prescribed drugs like my brother was when he was diagnosed with diabetes 20 years later. What changed in one generation?

Every time that I needed encouragement, I always called my best friend Kathy. When we talked, I asked her why I was not more grateful for my recovery because, if I had gotten better sooner, I might not have made some business decisions that caused financial problems for my family. Kathy simply said, "You can get your money back."

My answer was, "I might be able to get my money back, but my time has been lost forever."

After a deep discussion, Kathy and I agreed that I had to go through a grieving process, which might take time. The anger did not go away overnight; I had to be purposeful about getting over my anger. I went back to reading my motivational books that I had relied on before and other books by Joel Osteen, a pastor at Lakewood Church in Houston, Texas. This helped and I still do this today when I find myself dwelling in the past.

I worked on calming myself down when I felt angry at myself for the impact that my disease had had on my family. I walked in my yard and worked in my garden. In addition, I carried mustard seeds in my pocket as a reminder of my faith, and focused on what I had gained, not what I had lost.

I felt better when I shared my story with others in order to help them. Also, I started to keep notes about my recovery, and wrote articles for publication so that I could spread the good news of a dietary treatment for MS. When these articles were published, I received many calls and emails from people wanting help. I often met them face-to-face, and sometimes even with their families to share my story. Furthermore, I spoke with groups of MS patients – hoping to have a positive impact on their recoveries. I did my best to spread the information that I thought was being withheld by a majority of the medical professionals. I was surprised that most patients had no knowledge about the dietary treatment with which others were having success.

When I realized that the information about recovery from MS (without the dangerous drugs.), was still a secret, the mission for this book was shaped. I started to blog on MS websites. I noticed that my comments about the drug treatment being dangerous and recommending the diet treatment were being deleted. In many cases, the drug companies control these sites as well.

Oftentimes on these MS websites, I received messages in which some called me a liar, and some said I was mis-diagnosed. Still others preferred to smoke marijuana while on disability. Unfortunately, I was discouraged by some of the patients' comments and I stopped blogging.

I learned a few lessons from my "pity party." First, "this too shall pass." Second, I learned that if I can cure my MS, I can do anything. However, I had to be patient with myself because, having been sick for so long, I was bound to have problems that could not be solved overnight. Again, I knew that I had to take control of my own destiny! This time, though, I was ready to restart my life with my next adventure! I was ready to dream big!

Dream big! Get your life back!

After Mother's Day 2008, and every day since, I religiously stayed on my gluten-free diet, and got better each day. The first sign of recovery was my energy level. Before, I had to "rest" for two hours in the middle of the day and be in bed by 8pm. Now, I could skip the rest time.

Next, my MS brain fog started to lift. My thinking was sharper, and my memory was better. My speech improved within a week – so much so that my friends noticed it while speaking with me on the phone. Jim also noticed my improvement.

My Husband's Account of My Recovery

I noticed that Debbie was doing well within days of going gluten-free. I was not skeptical. Understanding Celiac Disease, it seemed to me she would probably continue to improve by staying on the diet. I believed that Debbie was recovering because of the gluten-free diet. Her illness was stressful for me; however, Debbie's recovery lessened the stress on me. I would highly recommend that anyone suffering from symptoms similar to Debbie's to eliminate gluten from their diet to see if they get better.

My Daughter's Account of My Recovery

The day after she cut out gluten, she told me over the phone that she felt better. It was immediate. I was very happy that she was doing so much better. I was afraid that it might stop helping after a while, and that she would revert back.

I believe that she had severe Celiac Disease that was undiagnosed. I think the cause of most, or all of her health issues was Celiac Disease.

The main thing I realized was that doctors don't have all the answers. I would recommend that a person take their health into their own hands. Don't rely on doctors for all of the answers. Try a holistic approach. I would describe my mom as a very determined person.

My Sister's Account of My Recovery

I noticed my sister was doing well immediately. The day we were in the gardens in Montgomery County, she told me that she was feeling better, and I could also tell when we talked over the phone, but I really didn't think she was doing that well until we went to the park.

I can't remember how long it was until I went back, but it was after she had been gluten-free for about 10 or 11 months. I think I had gone up for Spring, but I remember how much more energy she had; she looked better, and she had color to her. We went to the gardens in Montgomery County and walked to the Arboretum. I remember sitting about halfway around and realizing how far and how long timewise we had walked – I remember telling Debbie – the last time I was there, she couldn't have done this. I would have been carrying her at that point.

We still visit Walt Disney Park! Now, we ride rides, run from one ride to the next, run to play Buzz again and run to catch the fireworks. That would never have happened before the "cure."

My Cousin's Account of My Recovery

It seems like the next time I talked to Debbie, she was saying that she had cured herself of MS. She had just decided that she was not going to take the medications, as the side effects were worse than the MS and would probably kill her. It was Mother's Day, and Debbie looked at Jennifer, her daughter, and said "I'm not having this. I am getting well!" And she did. In a fairly short time, maybe 6 months, she had changed her lifestyle and diet, and was feeling better.

We went out to lunch a few years later after she had written an article for a local journal about her success. She had noticed that she was gluten intolerant, and completely eliminated gluten from her diet. Debbie was much more energetic! She had boundless energy and she moved with a spring in her step. She was excited to share her news and become successful in real estate.

And then Debbie helped us sell Mom and Dad's house, driving hours away from her home on countless occasions, doing whatever it took from meetings with us, to inspections, and to an open house. I have watched Debbie work and am inspired by her can-do attitude and follow-through. She has as much or more energy than most people her age and appears to be in great health.

And now Debbie is writing a book so that others can cure themselves and improve their lives. I am so proud of her!

Who knew that, after much research on my own, I would discover a simple dietary treatment that would CURE my Multiple Sclerosis? Within just a few days, I started to feel better, and I began my journey to full recovery of my health! It was hard for me to believe that a simple dietary treatment could produce such monumental, gargantuan results!!!

My recovery was progressing steadily toward regaining my health, and I then had the confidence to start something new. I sold the part of my marketing business that I no longer wanted to do.

Getting my life back

I thought that it was a good idea to go back into government service – especially in an area in which I had extensive experience. I had read that if a person had a disability, they had a better chance of being hired by the government. To apply for a job as a disabled person required being certified by their doctor. I knew that this would be easy for me because of my MS diagnosis. I made an appointment to see my neurologist, whom I had not seen in two years.

When he came into the room to speak with me and to check my symptoms, he commented on how good I was doing. I told him that I had been on a gluten-free diet since May 2008. He told me he had another patient who was getting better on a gluten-free diet, too. I wondered if he had told his other MS patients about the success of such a diet, or was he still hooked only on prescribing drugs. He quickly added that I should be on the drugs. I asked him why. He did not respond directly; instead, he told me, "Your MS is not cured." I responded, "You don't have to call me cured, but, if all my symptoms are gone, that's good enough for me!"

In 2009 the job market was extremely limited. I had hoped that my disability status would help me get hired. I found a job that was similar to the one I had had earlier in my career when I worked at the NASA library. I submitted the application online, but also made an appointment to submit it in person. On the drive to the office, I quickly realized that I would not be able to work a 9 to 5 job because the commute – an hour each way on a good day – would not be possible for my body. However, I kept my appointment and turned in my application, but I was not offered the job. I would not have accepted it if I had been selected. I also did not want to have to ask for disability accommodations, which I would have had to have after such a long commute.

On the drive home, I confirmed my idea that I must remain self-employed because I needed to have full control of my time. Therefore, I decided to pursue a career as a real estate agent. I had always wanted to have a career in real estate, and now the timing was perfect. My children were on their own and I was recovering my health. When I got home, I called a friend who was an agent. She told me that I had to take classes, and then pass a state test; I signed up for the classes that day.

When I arrived at the first class, I said a little prayer of thanks. An unbelievable feeling of power came over me – given how far I had come in such a short time. In one year, I had gone from planning for my family after my death from MS, to being healthy enough to start a new career. During the first class, I was amazed how clearly I was thinking, and how I could remember every new thing that I was learning. I finished the class on time, passed all the class tests, and passed the state test on the first try! In August 2009 I became a real estate agent.

When I joined Coldwell Banker, I was named "Rookie of the Year" for my outstanding work ethic and the numerous clients I was able to help with their real estate needs.

DEBBIE MCGRANN

HOPE

"I don't think of all the misery, but of
the beauty that still remains."
Anne Frank

"Let your hopes, not your hurts,
shape your future."
Robert H. Schuller

"God sends the dawn that we might see
the might-have-beens that still might be."
Robert Brault

CHAPTER SEVEN

The Answer to My Medical Mystery

Meeting Dr. Fasano

In January 2009, I still owned a marketing business in which I visited my clients at the start of the year to discuss business planning. When I met with my client Mary, she commented on how much better I looked since she had seen me a few months before. She knew about my MS, and previously we had discussed my progress. Like most people I meet, she had a family member with MS, and questioned me about my health issues. She asked what I was doing to get better. I explained my gluten-free dietary treatment. She told me that one of her employees was also having great success with her health on a gluten-free diet. She called her employee Melissa into our meeting to introduce us.

Melissa was wonderful about sharing her story of recovery with me. She told me the specifics of the gluten-free diet that was helping her with her previously undiagnosed Celiac Disease. She also raved about her doctor, Dr. Alessio Fasano. She told me that he was a pediatric gastroenterologist, and an expert in Celiac Disease. She also said that he was local and was accepting new patients. I was so grateful for her help and for this new information.

At the time, Dr. Fasano was professor of pediatrics, medicine, and physiology, and director of the Mucosal Biology Research Center, as well as the Center for Celiac Research at the University of Maryland School of Medicine. I made an appointment with him but had to wait a few months due to his long client appointment list. While I waited for my appointment, I did some research on Dr. Fasano, and discovered that he had written an article, "Surprises from Celiac Disease," which was published in the journal *Scientific American* in August 2009. I went to my local library and made a copy of the article. I was amazed to see his scientific research that proved that my MS was caused by my undiagnosed Celiac Disease. Here was the missing link to my autoimmune disease.

When I got to my appointment with Dr. Fasano, I was surprised that I was in a pediatric waiting room filled with children's books, toys and furniture. I felt a little out of place.

When I was put in an examination room, a nurse came in, introduced herself, and asked me if I would share my medical information and be part of their research study. Of course, I gave my permission – anything to help others with autoimmune issues. She also asked me if I would be willing to go back to eating gluten so that I could be tested for Celiac Disease. I told her that I would let her know after my discussion with Dr. Fasano. Mentally, I was reluctant to agree to disrupt my recovery by purposely eating gluten.

Dr. Fasano arrived right on time. I told him that his nurse had asked me if I would go back on gluten so I could be tested for Celiac Disease. He said, "Since you have been on a gluten-free diet for months, and you have recovered your health, testing was unnecessary. You have Celiac Disease." I thought, "Finally, a doctor with some common sense!"

In preparation for my appointment, I had prepared a one-page summary of my symptoms and family history. On the bottom of the page, I had the question, "Do I have MS, Celiac Disease, or both?"

He reviewed the summary I had prepared for him. When he got to the end, he looked at me and said, "You have Celiac Disease, and Celiac Disease **CAUSED** your MS." I was stunned and thrilled at the same time! Here was a world expert on Celiac Disease who had just told me the answer to my medical mystery, and reaffirmed that a gluten-free diet was indeed the cure for my MS. I was so happy. I then knew that I could continue with my gluten-free diet with the rock-solid knowledge that it was the answer to my recovery. My search for answers was over! Case closed!

CONCLUSION

My Multiple Sclerosis was **CAUSED** by undiagnosed Celiac Disease, and a gluten-free diet was the **ONLY** cure for Celiac Disease; therefore, a gluten-free diet was the cure for my Multiple Sclerosis, and the diet was working to restore my health!

Celiac Disease – An Introduction

Background of Dr. Fasano

There are several leading experts on Celiac Disease; however, the premier expert is Dr. Alessio Fasano. Currently, Dr. Fasano is Vice Chair of Basic Translational, and Clinical Research and Division Chief of Pediatric Gastroenterology and Nutrition at the Mass General Hospital for Children in Boston, Massachusetts. Dr. Fasano also serves on the Board for the Celiac Disease Foundation.

Background of the Problem

According to Dr. Fasano, when humans discovered seeds, they began to grow crops for various purposes. As a result, civilizations began to experiment with various types of seeds to create blends of wheat, barley, and rye. Although seeds provided geographic stability to groups of people because they no longer had to travel far to get their food, an unintended consequence of such a stable food supply was creation of the disease known as Celiac Disease. Celiac Disease is a malabsorption disease that occurs when people eat gluten, which is a protein that is found in rye, wheat, and barley. Gluten is a relatively new problem that occurred due to the stabilization of crops. Unfortunately, gluten had devastating effects on small intestines, and these effects generally start in childhood.

Today, scientists understand that Celiac Disease has a genetic component, and is an autoimmune disease. As a result, the effects are that people with Celiac Disease often experience diarrhea and abdominal pain. Moreover, Celiac Disease develops in the small intestines, which become abnormal as a result of extended exposure to gluten.

Discovery of the Problem

In 1887, a British doctor named Samuel Gee discovered Celiac Disease. He observed that Celiac Disease occurred due to a persistent problem of food ingestion. He noted that it affected people of all ages, but especially children. Although he knew that Celiac Disease was a disease which had something to do with food ingestion and dietary choices, he still incorrectly prescribed that kids should eat thinly sliced toast.

After World War II, a Dutch pediatrician, Willem-Karel Dicke, noticed that the mortality rate of children in the Netherlands went from 35% to zero due to a shortage of bread. However, once the scarcity of bread disappeared and bread consumption returned to normal levels, the rate of deaths due to Celiac Disease went to their previous levels. This led to other scientists to correctly identify gluten as the primary culprit. This insight helped scientists discover that repeated exposure to gluten-containing products damages the structure of villi in the small intestines – the villi becoming abnormally large.

Prevalence of the Problem - The Leaky Gut Theory

Researchers studying Celiac Disease have made several important discoveries. One is that an enzyme (transglutaminase) makes it easy to detect Celiac Disease. Apparently, this enzyme, and/or antibodies to it, leak out of the intestines and into the abdomen to heal the small intestines. The presence of this enzyme has allowed researchers to easily identify those with Celiac Disease.

Dr. Fasano and his team went on a hunt to find those who were affected by Celiac Disease. They found that 1 in 133 people were affected by Celiac Disease, which meant that the disease was more common than previously reported. They also discovered that, although more people are now known to be affected by the disease, the symptoms may not be as extreme if only a small part of the intestines is impacted. However, the most important discovery is that, because Celiac Disease is a malabsorption disease, that prevents the proper absorption of nutrients, it can also be the root cause of many other autoimmune diseases, such as; osteoporosis, epilepsy, lupus, MS, etc.

As a result of gluten research, other autoimmune diseases can be studied as well. Dr. Fasano's research has identified three factors that underlie Celiac Disease. One of the factors is an environmental trigger that is within wheat, barley, and rye – called gluten. The second characteristic is one's genes. In most people the third characteristic is indigestible gluten fragments, which often leak into the gut through microscopic junctions. Past researchers did not study these junctions in the gut because doctors had been taught that it was rare for anything to leak out of the intestines because they were "built like a pipe."

Recovery

I noticed that I was getting better at home. I did not have to rest as much. I was less confused. My speech was better, and I had more energy. Within days of starting my gluten-free diet, I asked members of my family and some friends what they thought. My son-in-law thought that I never had MS, and that I had been misdiagnosed.

My friends noticed my voice was stronger. Clearly, the only variable that I had changed in my life was the switch to a gluten-free diet. I know that there are people who think that I have not been cured. However, when people say that to me, I like to refer them to the definition of a cure:

> Let me remind you of the meaning of the noun **cure**:
> 1. A method or course of medical treatment.
> 2. Restoration of health.

After starting my gluten-free diet in May 2008, I started to think that I was going to be OK. The year 2009 turned out to be a very pivotal year. My daughter Jennifer and her husband Jason were expecting their first child on March 10. We knew the exact date because it was going to be a caesarian delivery. This would also be our first grandchild! Of course, we were all very excited!

This pending event reminded me of a time in 2008 before I started my gluten-free diet. Jim and I attended the baptism of our friend's first grandchild. I was so weak that I was afraid to hold the baby while standing up. I had to sit down in a chair, and my friend handed me the baby. I still was having trouble holding the baby safely, so I passed him to Jim. It made me sad to think that I would never be able to hold my own grandchildren, much less play with them or walk to the playground with them.

When the delivery date was getting close, I asked Jennifer if she wanted me to plan to stay and help her and Jason with the baby. She said that she and Jason would like to handle it themselves. I respected their decision. However, I knew that, as new parents, they were going to need help. I thought that she didn't want to ask me to help because she didn't know if I would be up to it physically. Jennifer and Jason lived out of our state, and they didn't see me often. Maybe she was afraid that she would be taking care of a new baby and me, too. I packed enough clothes to be able to spend a week with them if they changed their minds.

On March 10, 2009, Ella was born: a perfect, beautiful, healthy baby girl! All of us were so excited! However, during the delivery, the doctor accidentally nicked Jennifer's bladder (he was talking on his cell phone), which caused her to have a longer recovery, and prevented her from going up and down stairs. Jason spent the first night in the hospital with Jennifer and Ella.

In the morning, they both asked me to stay longer. The reality of a new baby was setting in quickly. Of course, I knew that it would. I had the honor and privilege of spending a week taking care of Ella so that Jennifer and Jason could rest as much as possible with a fussy baby. I cooked meals for them and took care of their dog. I felt so blessed that I was healthy enough to help them and spend this special time with my first grandchild. I celebrated my 55th birthday with them on March 17, 2009. It was hard to believe that I had gotten this much better, so fast – what a blessing!

Support Groups

While I was struggling with my MS symptoms, I did not attend any support groups. For me, talking about my symptoms was not therapeutic; it made me feel worse and hopeless.

In 2009, I had been on my gluten-free diet for a year, and was feeling much, much better. I was convinced from my research that my recovery would continue. After I discovered Dr. Fasano's article on the connection between MS and Celiac Disease, I was empowered to spread the wonderful news of my recovery, as well as the science that supported a gluten-free diet as, by far, the best treatment for MS. I called the leader of a local MS support group to ask him how many people usually attended the meetings. I made copies of Dr. Fasano's article, "Surprises from Celiac Disease," and more information that I had discovered that I thought would help others understand the connection between MS recovery and a gluten-free diet. I made copies for everyone at the meeting. This group was advertised as "newly diagnosed" MS patients.

When I arrived at the meeting, I discovered that ALL of the attendees were on one or more drugs for MS. The meeting was facilitated by a representative of the MS Society. There were about 20 MS patients, plus their caregivers, at the meeting. The attendees went around the table introducing themselves and saying which drugs they were currently taking.

When it was my turn to speak, I introduced myself as a "recovered MS patient." I described my MS symptoms. I also told them that I had never taken any drugs and had been cured by a gluten-free diet alone. I handed out all the information that I had brought for them to read. The room was dead silent after my presentation.

The group leader (from the MS Society) interrupted the silence with the statement, "The MS Society does not recognize any diet as a treatment for MS." She then went on to say, "I am 61 years old and happy with where I am with my drug therapy." She was strapped into her chair so that she could sit up straight. She needed help getting from the chair to her walker. She was very pale and thin. I couldn't help but wonder if her drugs were really working. I was in MUCH better shape than she was, and, of course, with NO drugs! At the time, I was only a few years younger than she was.

For the rest of the meeting, no one spoke to me. No one asked me any questions about my gluten-free diet. No one called me after the meeting after they had had time to review the information that I had given them. I was surprised at the lack of curiosity. As I drove home, I reflected on how grateful and excited I would have been to get that information when I was first diagnosed! It saddened me to think that these patients were so influenced by this leader's blatantly incorrect and biased opinion.

It seemed obvious that the pharmaceutical companies had infiltrated the support groups. I never attended another MS group.

DEBBIE MCGRANN

UNSTOPPABLE

"The best way to predict your future is to create it."
Abraham Lincoln

"The question isn't who is going to let me;
it's who is going to stop me."
Ayn Rand

"Nothing is impossible. The word itself says
'I'M POSSIBLE'!"
Audrey Hepburn

CHAPTER EIGHT

My New Normal

Communicating My New Life to Family and Friends

When I discovered that I had Celiac Disease, I was diagnosed by Dr. Fasano. I did not know as much about Celiac Disease as I know now. Yet, I needed to explain to my family and friends what Celiac Disease was all about. Therefore, I started to research and read everything I could get my hands on just to explain to them what was going on in my body. I knew that some of my family members and friends were interested, but I needed to know a lot more about Celiac Disease so that I could better explain everything to them. Listed below are a few of the questions that those around me asked, and how I phrased and framed my answers to them.

Question: *What is Celiac Disease?*
Answer: Celiac disease is an autoimmune disease that causes those who have a genetic predisposition to have difficulty absorbing certain vitamins and minerals via their small intestines. It is commonly

referred to as a "malabsorption disease," as well as a "leaky gut" disease because eating gluten products can cause harm to the intestines that may have disastrous health effects over time – causing various other diseases, such as MS, autism, diabetes, etc.

Question: *What does it mean to be gluten-free?*
Answer: This means that I cannot eat any foods whatsoever that contain gluten. Foods that have gluten mainly include wheat, barley, and rye – which can damage not only small intestines, but also immune systems. Some of my friends and family members were concerned that I was not eating enough and offered me foods that they knew contained gluten. When I declined, they replied, "A little won't hurt you." On one occasion, when my husband Jim was with me, he emphasized that a little bit could actually kill me!

Question: *Does this mean you can never eat at restaurants?*
Answer: No. I can still eat at restaurants. However, I have to be careful about what I order. Most restaurants have gluten-free items on their menus. How the food is cooked in the kitchen is also important. For example, I always ask the manager if the French fries are fried in the same fryer as the breaded foods, which would cause cross contamination. There are usually standard items that I can eat like fruits, vegetables, and meats.

Although restaurants are getting better, they still have a lot to learn about their gluten-free guests. One of the reasons I enjoy going to Disney World is that they are extremely prepared for gluten-free guests. It makes me feel very comfortable eating there. I visit Disney World as much as possible. It's my "happy place for food!"

Question: *Will your health improve after going on a gluten-free diet?*
Answer: My health improved remarkably after I started my gluten-free diet. Furthermore, much research proves that eating a gluten-free diet helps me stay alive and well – hopefully to live a normal life

span. My numbness went away, my pain subsided, my ADHD improved, and I was more focused! Also, my allergies became less severe. I even have two pet cats!

Question: *How soon did you notice that your health was improving as a result of being on a gluten-free diet?*
Answer: I noticed it immediately. I used to have "brain fog" every day. When I woke up the first morning after starting my gluten-free diet, my "brain fog" had lifted. I couldn't believe this was possible. I referred to the book, *Gluten-free for Dummies*, in which it states that some patients experience immediate results. I was thrilled!

Question: *What is more important, taking a supplement to help gluten sensitivity or avoiding foods which contain gluten?*
Answer: It is more important to solve your malabsorption problem first; by not eating any gluten products. This is what is preventing you from getting the nutrients and minerals your body needs from the food you eat. What you stop eating (gluten) is more important than supplements you take to help with whatever ails you.

Would Your Doctor Lie to You?

Trust. We are supposed to be able to trust our doctors' advice. They are only concerned about the wellbeing of their patients, right? Would YOUR doctor(s) lie to you? Mine did!

As of July 2008, I had been on my gluten-free diet since May 2008, I had gotten much better, but I still had work to do on my path to full recovery. My main focus was my severe osteoporosis. I had been referred to an endocrinologist.

I was so excited to talk to this doctor because I was confident that she would put all the parts of my medical puzzle together for me. I gathered all my medical records together and headed off to my appointment, arriving 30 minutes early. As she entered the room, I jumped up to shake her hand, and told her how glad I was to be there. She looked a little taken aback. I then explained that I had been ill for a long time and had been to many specialists. I felt that she was finally the right specialist to help me get better!

We reviewed my medical history. I told her that I was on a gluten-free diet, was feeling much better, and my MS symptoms were lessening. I told her that I probably had Celiac Disease. She asked me what I knew about the blood test for Celiac Disease. I told her that the testing for Celiac Disease is not reliable if the patient is already on a gluten-free diet. Nonetheless, she gave me the order for the blood testing, including the test for Celiac Disease.

On my second visit, I again arrived early. and was shown into an examination room where I laid out the results of all the tests that the doctor had ordered. A nurse arrived and was relieved that I had all my test results – because they had not yet received their copies. She asked to borrow MY reports to copy for the doctor. Obviously, the doctor had not reviewed my test results before this visit; fortunately, I had reviewed everything.

My Best Friend Kathy's Account

I am a professional organizer. I thought I was pretty organized before Debbie's illness and recovery, but Debbie's experiences with her various doctors taught me that I have to be my own "general contractor" when it comes to my healthcare. I have organized my own medical records and take them with me whenever I visit a new doctor. I've also taught classes on organizing medical records, using Debbie's experiences as an example of why it's so important. I also wrote a chapter in my book, My Journey to an Organized Life (Katherine Trezise), about organizing medical records. I have been taking cholesterol medication for many years. My cholesterol levels are now excellent, and I've been able to decrease the dosage. Recently I asked my doctor if I could get off the medicine completely since one of its side effects is dementia. She said yes, BUT I would have to make certain diet and exercise changes. I probably would never have even asked that question had it not been for Debbie's illness and recovery.

The doctor announced that my osteoporosis had gotten worse. She immediately suggested (with great glee, I noticed) that I should take the drug Reclast. I asked her for the chemical name, and I asked her how to spell it. She seemed annoyed at this request. I told her that this drug sounded a lot like Fosamax.

I asked her if Reclast had been tested on MS patients. She did not know. I asked her if Reclast had been tested on Celiac Disease patients. She said, "You don't have Celiac Disease." I reminded her that the testing was flawed because I had already started my gluten-free diet. Why was she misleading me about having Celiac Disease? I told her that on the commercial for Reclast, it said it was not to be used on patients with low calcium. She said, "You don't have low calcium." Here is where she was wrong again. The results for my test for low calcium were not included in the test results that she had (I had provided her the results, and she had obviously not reviewed them). Why would she lie to me about my test results? She was advising me to take a drug that had serious possible side effects without the proper testing on patients like me. Why? I suspect that there were some very strong financial incentives for doctors who prescribed this new drug.

I reminded her of my horrible reaction to Fosamax. I told her that I took Fosamax once a week, and that this new drug that she was suggesting is taken once a year. "That seems about 50 times stronger to me," I said.

She explained, "It is stronger, but it is a different delivery system." Reclast is given by infusion in a hospital. I replied, "It sounds like it will kill me 50 times quicker." She was really mad at this point. My persistence and curiosity were obviously bothering her. She said, "I can see you are afraid to take this drug." I replied, "I'm not afraid, I just think it's a bad idea." With an angry wave of her hand, she said, "Then get out!" I was being thrown out of a doctor's office for asking too many questions! I was trying to protect myself from her bad advice!

I gathered my test results and left. When I got home, I did some quick research on Reclast. I told my husband Jim how bad the side effects were. Our opinion was that I would have had a very bad outcome had I taken her advice.

> **"First, do no harm"**
> **Hippocratic Oath**

Would the pharmaceutical companies lie to you?

As I write this book in 2019, drug company executives, doctors, pain management executives, drug store managers, etc. are being arrested and charged with illegal drug trafficking. In my opinion (and those of many others, too), they are worse than the drug dealers on the streets! They use their positions as trusted professionals to get patients addicted to pain medications! They created an epidemic of abuse in which over 70,000 people, mostly young adults, died in 2017. Government oversight failed to protect patients from the pharmaceutical companies. Beware of people, including your doctor, who, too often, put profits over patient health. Do your own research. Trust, but verify.

NUTRITION

"The doctor of the future will give no medication, but will interest his patients in the care of the human frame, diet and in the cause and prevention of disease."
Thomas A. Edison

"The man who uses intelligence with respect to his diet, his sleeping habits and who exercises properly, is beyond any question of doubt taking the very best preventive medicines provided so freely and abundantly by nature."
Joseph Pilates

"The person who takes medicine must recover TWICE, once from the disease and once from the medicine."
William Osler, MD.

CHAPTER NINE

Drugs or No Drugs

MS Drugs vs. Gluten-free Diet: What Would You Do?

When I was diagnosed with Multiple Sclerosis in 2001, the only treatment option I was given involved strong drugs with many undesirable side effects. I chose not to take the drugs. Since they do not claim to cure Multiple Sclerosis, I thought the side effects were not worth the risks.

Here are some of the most common Multiple Sclerosis drugs and their side effects:

Avonex, Betaseron, and **Copaxone** are commonly referred to as the ABC drugs. These are strong interferon drugs taken every-other-day or weekly by injection. Side effects include depression; flu-like symptoms; liver, heart, blood, and thyroid problems; and the risk of miscarriage, and seizures.

Tysabri increases your chances of getting a rare brain infection that usually causes death or severe disability. This infection is called progressive multifocal leukoencephalopathy (PML). There is no known treatment, prevention, or cure for PML.

These side effects seem worse than the disease. Patients today, more than ten years later, are still being pushed toward drug therapy only! Are there any other options available? My treatment option is a life-long gluten-free diet. After being on the diet for a short time (months), all of my Multiple Sclerosis symptoms were relieved. I was on my way to a complete recovery! Do the MS drugs have the same success? No!!!

Here are some of the most common side effects of a gluten-free diet: **NONE**!

Are the drugs and bankruptcy worth dying for?

When I was trying to decide whether to take the MS drugs or not, I had to consider the financial costs to my family. In 2017, the cost of MS drug treatments was estimated to exceed $70,000 dollars a year! I reasoned that I was not going to take the drugs for a variety of reasons: I did not think it was worth the risk of the side effects, one of which is death by PML. The drugs are not a cure. The drug company's own information claims, "You MAY not get worse." I have seen NO evidence of a single MS patient recovering their health while on any of these drugs. I was not willing to give up the time to go to the hospital and get the infusions.

I was not willing to be sick for days after the infusions (with "flu like symptoms"). Even with the best health insurance available, the cost of this drug would bankrupt most MS patients and their families. To me, the risks and the costs were too high.

Calculating the Cost

The cost of the drugs was a consideration for my husband and me. At the time, our daughter was in college, and our son was a senior in high school and looking at colleges. Our family finances were OK, but these extra costs would have been a burden that I did not think we could bear without hardships to our family. Also, I did not want to bankrupt my family for drugs that clearly would not be helpful to my recovery.

My husband and I discussed the situation. We both agreed that if these drugs were the cure for my MS, we would do whatever it took to pay for them. We would sell the house, we would cash in our retirement accounts, and whatever it would take we would do. However, the drug information only said the drugs "may" help stop progression of my symptoms. That was not good enough for me. I told my husband that I would not agree to the drug therapy. I think my husband was very worried about my decision, but he supported me 100%.

Tysabri – A Case Study

This book started as a series of articles I wrote and published in a local woman's health journal. I received many phone calls and emails requesting more information and help. I did what I could. I met with a few people and shared my story. I also spoke at a few wellness centers offering classes for MS patients. However, at the time, I was not in a position to offer much assistance. I was trying to develop my real estate business. Also, I had not done enough research to feel confident to offer extensive advice.

I still felt the need to share my story of recovery with other MS patients to give them hope and another option beyond drugs. I started posting on MS websites and Facebook pages. I was surprised and disheartened by the strong negative reactions I was receiving. I started to avoid discussing my recovery.

One day I received an email from a mother telling me that her daughter was diagnosed with MS at age 21. She was advised to start on the MS drugs immediately. She started taking Tysabri. She was dead at age 29! This mother told me to keep warning people about the dangers of the MS drugs. This mother was the motivation that I needed to complete this book. I am sorry that I do not have her contact information. I hope this book finds its way to her.

The following article was so riveting to me that I felt it necessary to repeat it in its entirety.

Death and Dividends: The Tysabri Debacle

For the last three to four years, neurologists have been talking about the coming of a much more effective drug for MS. That drug was first called Antegren and then Tysabri. The story of Tysabri illustrates some risky and unsavory aspects of the search for an effective drug for MS.

Tysabri is a humanized, monoclonal antibody that is produced by transgenic goats in their milk. A monoclonal antibody is a designer drug that targets one specific protein in the body, and basically knocks it out of action. MS research has led to the concept that MS is driven by activated T cells that are sensitized to myelin. Such autoreactive T cells are activated in the blood mainly through an immune encounter with a foreign protein from an infectious agent or food. The activated, myelin aggressive T cells then migrate to the brain, pass through the blood-brain barrier, and lead an attack on the myelin. It was reasoned that if a drug could stop or greatly hinder the passage of these auto aggressive T cells across a blood-brain barrier, then the MS disease process could be substantially short-circuited. Activated T cells cross a blood-brain barrier by sticking on the blood vessel wall, and then pushing through it. A monoclonal antibody, which was to become Tysabri, was developed to knock out the protein on the T cells (VLA-4) that allows them to stick on the blood vessel wall.

Preliminary studies indicated that Tysabri was seemingly safe over the short term with a few bad allergic reactions being the only notable adverse effect. By 2001, Elan and Biogen, the drug companies which were producing Tysabri, predicted billions of dollars in future revenue and their stocks started to soar. The Phase III trial began in late 2002 and, after only one year, the companies applied to the Food and Drug Administration (FDA) in the USA to approve the drug even though there wasn't any evidence that it slowed disease progression. At the same time the drug was also tested for Crohn's Disease, a gastrointestinal autoimmune disease, but was found to have no significant effect. One person on Tysabri in the Crohn's trial died of apparent brain cancer.

In November of 2004 the FDA approved Tysabri for use based on the first-year result of fewer attacks and MRI-detected lesions, and, soon afterward, neurologists were infusing their patients with this new, very expensive drug. The company's stocks climbed to new heights.

The last two weeks of February 2005 were very eventful. On February 14 Biogen director, Robert Pangia, sold 15,570 shares for a profit of $954,844. On Feb 15, Biogen's executive chairman, William Rastetter, sold more than 120,000 shares, yielding a $7.45-million profit. On February 18 Thomas Bucknum, a Biogen executive vice president and the company's general counsel, sold 89,700 shares for a profit of $1.9 million. Later that same day, Biogen informed the FDA that one Tysabri patient had died of a very rare brain disease known as PML (progressive multifocal leukoencephalopathy), and that another patient also likely had the disease.

PML occurs when the JC virus, which most people carry, rises from a dormant state due to a weakened immune system, and destroys the myelin in the brain at a very rapid rate. PML is a very ugly disease which usually ends in death over a few months. Given that Tysabri prevents T cells from entering the brain, and thus reduces immunological control of the JC virus, it is extremely likely that it is the main cause of the PML.

On February 27, Elan and Biogen issued a glowing press release describing the results of the two-year Tysabri clinical trials. It sounded like the promised drug had arrived. On February 28 the FDA issued a terse statement stating that two Tysabri patients had PML and that the drug was being voluntarily withdrawn from use by Elan and Biogen. Both stocks fell like rocks with Elan losing 60% of its value and Biogen 40%. When questioned about the executives who had possibly made illegal stock trades, Biogen, stated "All these trades preceded that quick and decisive action, which was guided exclusively by concern for patient safety and our commitment to the MS community." The Securities Exchange Commission will likely investigate whether insider-trading laws were violated.

Throughout most of March it was widely agreed that Tysabri would likely make a comeback as early as the fall. Then at the end of March came the news that the patient in the Crohn's/Tysabri study who had supposedly died of cancer had died of PML. As I write this, they are still debating whether Tysabri will be brought back despite its potentially fatal side effects.

There are several incidents connected with the Tysabri saga that need clarification. It is surprising the Biogen doctors misdiagnosed PML as brain cancer in 2003, especially when PML is a possibility with any drug that has a major effect on the immune system of the brain. Also, it is unclear why it took at least a month after the PML cases were identified in the Tysabri and MS trials for the drug's withdrawal to be announced. This delay put many people at great risk. Furthermore, is it just coincidence that the Biogen executives unloaded their stock during this questionable delay? It is also surprising that Elan and Biogen put out a press release saying how fantastic Tysabri is, knowing full well that the next day the FDA was going announce the suspension of the drug because of ties to a deadly brain disease. And why did the FDA approve Tysabri after only one year of the Phase III trial given the potential of long-term side effects of such a powerful drug as well as the less than stellar results. These are all troubling questions without answers.

Persons with MS should realize that participating in a clinical trial is somewhat like playing Russian Roulette and that a drug company's desire for maximum profits may compromise their efforts to ensure maximum protection against harm. Drugs that short-circuit the immune system have bad side effects and death is always a possibility. Copaxone and the beta-interferon drugs are cakewalks compared to what is coming down the pipe. The drug companies know that any new "blockbuster" drug, such as Tysabri, must be significantly more effective than the current drugs and that means they will likely be much more damaging to the immune system.

I always find it incredible that many people recently diagnosed with MS will choose a potentially deadly drug over nutritional strategies that are completely safe and likely more effective. Luckily there are still some people with common sense who do not allow themselves to be sacrificed for profit.

This article was adapted in its entirety from www.direct-ms.org. This website was developed by Ashton Embry, Ph.D. and families with MS. The initial goal of the website was to search for the causes of MS, thereby, devising therapies which are nutrition based. Dr. Embry is a research scientist. His son, Matt (www.mshope.org) developed Multiple Sclerosis and he decided to comb the research literature on MS. Mr. Embry discovered that nutritional strategies play a significant role in the possible cure of MS.

DEBBIE MCGRANN

FOOD

"Leave your drugs in the chemist's pot if you can heal the patient with food."
Hippocrates

"Just as food causes chronic disease, it can be the most powerful cure."
Hippocrates

"To do nothing is sometimes a good remedy."
Hippocrates

CHAPTER TEN

Embarking on a Gluten-free Diet
Gluten-free Diet as the Cure for Celiac Disease

Can a diet cure disease? Can your diet cause your illness? Can a diet be a treatment for Multiple Sclerosis and the over 100 known autoimmune diseases? Hard to believe, but it is true. It was true for me and it may be true for you. It is certainly worth a try.

A gluten-free diet has been the only cure for Celiac Disease since 1950. Specifically, a gluten-free diet literally means food without wheat, barley, and rye. To be on a truly gluten-free diet requires that a person not eat the following categories of food:

- Bread
- Cereals
- Flours
- Pasta
- Cakes
- Biscuits
- And any sauces that are devised from wheat, rye, and/or barley.

I recommend that a person starting a gluten-free diet should only eat foods that are naturally occurring, such as meat, fruits, vegetables and eggs instead of buying the more expensive processed gluten-free foods. However they are available to you if you are willing to spend the extra money.

It is important that you thoroughly educate yourself about the foods that you can and cannot eat.

When you suffer from Celiac Disease, maintaining a gluten-free diet is critical to your success. It is important that, when you are traveling through the grocery aisles, that you stay on the outside aisles. Avoid all processed foods unless it is clearly labeled as "gluten-free." I recommend the book, *Gluten-free for Dummies*; that book gave me all the guidance that I needed to get started, and to proceed to master this new lifestyle.

Initially, following a gluten-free diet may be difficult, but I believe that you will see the results you desire. The most important key is to keep it simple. I do not recommend going on another diet, such as the caveman's diet, ketosis diet, or any other diet.

Starting a gluten-free diet gave me the immediate results that I had been seeking in a cure. This is why I know that I was cured.

> Let me remind you of the meaning of the noun **cure**:
> 1. A method or course of medical treatment.
> 2. Restoration of health.

I believe that I was given my life back when I started this diet, and, if you follow the diet, I pray that you will obtain the same results.

DEBBIE MCGRANN

GLUTEN-FREE SHOPPING GUIDE

Shop the Outer Rim

MAGAZINES	FROZEN FOODS	DAIRY & EGGS
CHECKOUT	SODA/PROCESSED FOODS	MEATS
	CLEANING ITEMS	
	BAKING ITEMS	
	CANNED FOOD	
FLOWERS & GIFTS	VEGETABLES FRUITS UNPROCESSED FOODS	CHEESE/YOGHURT ICE CREAM

Tips for starting a Gluten-free Diet Treatment

Before you begin your gluten-free dietary treatment, you must prepare yourself. Like me, you may encounter resistance from friends and family. You must be committed and have facts available to explain to your doubters the importance of this diet to your health. Remember, awareness of the gluten-free diet treatment is low. You have to be prepared to educate others, so be strong in your decision. The following are some tips to help you:

Educate yourself. Facts about the diet will give you confidence in yourself. My grocery store gives free tours with a dietician for their customers on special diets. Take advantage of this at your store.

Have reasonable expectations. I noticed an improvement overnight. However, that is not common. It usually takes weeks for most people to notice any improvement. Do not get discouraged if it takes longer to see results!

Remove all of the non-diet approved foods from your house. If you are in charge of the meals for you and your family, make it easy at the beginning. Make simple gluten-free meals for the entire family. This is what I do. I also avoid the gluten-free packaged foods. Instead, I focus on naturally gluten-free foods: fruit, vegetables, meat, and eggs. I avoid dairy and soy. Also, it does not bother me if my husband eats bread with his meal. Remember, keep it simple.

It is important that you check food labels because there may be hidden glutens in certain foods. It is also important to avoid malt liquors and beers.

Pick a date to start. I like the idea of picking a meaningful date, such as a birthday, an anniversary, or a holiday. I started my treatment on Mother's Day. Every year, I enjoy celebrating my recovery on that day. My celebration is usually just a quiet prayer of thanks, but I like taking the time to reflect on how far I have come. If you are starting a gluten-free diet for a child, I suggest starting when school is out, so that you have total control. Once school starts, make sure that the school knows your child's dietary needs.

Stay the course! This treatment may seem difficult at first. But if you keep it simple, it gets easier. There are NO side effects to this treatment! I think that once you start feeling better, you will never go back to eating gluten.

General Foods to Eat When on a Gluten-free Diet

I know that a gluten-free diet helped me to recover from the ravages of MS. I have learned that there are some foods that should be eaten on a gluten-free diet, and those that should be avoided. The foods that everyone can eat are meat, eggs, fruits and vegetables of all kinds. This should be easy to follow, because most of these foods are in the outer aisles of a grocery store. The good news about eating a lot of fruits and vegetables is that fruits and vegetables also contain a number of important, and even critical, minerals and vitamins. Hence, this will help Celiac patients to attain the level of nutrition that they need to live healthier lives.

The second group of foods to eat for Celiac patients are healthy fats like avocados and coconuts; you may also eat nuts and seeds - like walnuts, sunflower seeds, hemp and chia seeds. Lastly, beans and legumes are also good for a gluten-free diet. As mentioned above, most grocery stores carry "prepared" gluten-free products; however, some of these products can be very expensive.

PREVENTION

"An ounce of prevention is worth a pound of cure."
Benjamin Franklin

"After I was diagnosed with Celiac Disease, I said yes to food, with great enthusiasm. . ... I vowed to taste everything I could eat, rather than focusing on what I could not."
Shauna James Ahern

"Perhaps most important to keep in mind, however, is that it can be impossible to distinguish between the symptoms of MS and those of gluten sensitivity."
Shari Lieberman

CHAPTER ELEVEN

The Future of Celiac Disease

Why is Celiac Disease Increasing?

The old adage, "which came first the chicken or the egg?" is often discussed when studying why Celiac Disease is increasing. Several researchers have observed that the effects of Celiac Disease may actually be referring to what we call wheat breeding. Although the scope of this book is not prepared to discuss this in detail, I do believe that it is important to be aware of some of the recent research. The researchers looked at datasets of the 20th and 21st centuries to observe the evolution of wheat – starting 10,000 years ago.

Researchers at the *Journal of Agricultural and Food Chemistry* found that there is no corroborative evidence that wheat breeding is causing or has a relationship to the increased incidence of Celiac Disease. However, I think Celiac Disease is increasing due to the increase in consumption of processed foods. We need to go back to cooking at home using simple gluten-free ingredients. It takes some planning, but your health depends on it.

Attention Deficit Hyperactivity Disorder (ADHD)

Celiac Disease is a relatively new disease; however, there are several studies that show strong relationships between Celiac Disease and other major diseases or problems in our society. Once such link is the relationship between Celiac Disease and attention deficit hyperactivity disorder. I was diagnosed with ADHD by my neurologist soon after my MS diagnosis. I'm sure this is what caused all my trouble in school. I'm glad there were no drugs available to treat my ADHD!

Multiple Sclerosis (MS) and Celiac Disease

As I mentioned before, I was told by doctors that I had MS. Although the doctors had given me this label, I was determined in my spirit that I was going to overcome the symptoms of the disease and heal myself. I honestly did not know how, but I made up in my mind that I was going to do my best to cure myself regardless of the prognosis that the doctors had handed me.

Recently, researchers discovered that there is, in fact, a link between MS and Celiac Disease. I found this link quite by accident by telling everyone I knew about my illness (MS), and doing extensive library research.

As I mentioned earlier, I read a lot of the articles that Dr. Fasano has written, and this resulted in me changing my diet. In 2011, a study was reported in a BMC article, "Prevalence of Celiac Disease in MS Patients," which stated that MS patients were 5-10% more likely to have Celiac Disease. The study found that by placing MS patients on a gluten-free diet, they were able to lessen the effects of the MS symptoms. Thus, the research is very clear regarding the link between MS and Celiac Disease. I am eternally grateful for the research that is done in this area, and I would encourage those of you with auto-immune disorders to go on the gluten-free diet.

Autism

Definition from the Centers for Disease Control and Prevention (CDC)

Autism: A chronic developmental disorder usually diagnosed between 18 and 30 months of age. Symptoms include problems with social interaction and communication as well as repetitive interests and activities. At this time, the cause of autism is not known although many experts believe it to be a genetically based disorder that occurs before birth.

Could the genetically based disorder be Celiac Disease? Could the trigger be vaccines and/or gluten?

Multiple Sclerosis

Definition from the Centers for Disease Control and Prevention (CDC)

Multiple Sclerosis: (MS) is a disease of the central nervous system characterized by the destruction of the myelin sheath surrounding neurons, resulting in the formation of "plaques." MS is a progressive and usually fluctuation disease with exacerbations (patients feeling worse) and remissions (patients feeling better) over many decades. Eventually, in most patients, remissions do not reach baseline levels and permanent disability and sometimes death occurs. The cause of MS is unknown. The most widely held hypotheses is that MS occurs in patients with a genetic susceptibility and that some environmental factors "trigger" exacerbations. MS is 3 times more common in in women than men, with diagnosis usually made as young adults.

Could the genetic susceptibility be Celiac Disease? Could the trigger be vaccines and/or gluten? According to the CDC, your child should not receive live vaccines if he or she has a weakened immune system (Celiac Disease?). They advise parents to talk to their child's doctor to determine which vaccines your child can and cannot get at each visit, and how to protect your child's health.

Attention Parents:

It is up to you to protect your children from adverse reactions of vaccines. The pharmaceutical companies are not willing to admit that there can be any dangers from vaccines. Therefore, the doctors are not receiving any guidance on which children should not be given the "live vaccines." If you have any family history of any autoimmune diseases, your child should not be on the same vaccination schedule as other children.

Definition from the Centers for Disease Control and Prevention

Live vaccine: A vaccine in which live virus is weakened (attenuated) through chemical or physical processes in order to produce an immune response without causing severe effects of the disease. Attenuated vaccines currently licensed in the United States include measles, mumps, rubella, shingles (herpes zoster), varicella, and yellow fever.

Could it be that the live vaccine shot given to children is the "trigger" to autism in childhood, and/or developing MS later? It is interesting that most children diagnosed with autism are boys, and most young adults diagnosed with MS are women.

In my own family, my brother has what today would be diagnosed as autism. I remember my father saying, many times, that, "he was fine until he got that shot." My brother's son has Asperger's. I have multiple autoimmune diseases including MS. My daughter has gluten sensitivity. My son has ADD. My granddaughter had an adverse reaction to her MMR shot. The doctor had asked if there were any family members with autoimmune diseases. My daughter said yes, and she told the doctor that her mother had MS. The doctor took no precautions with Avery even knowing the family history. Did she not know the shot could be dangerous for Avery? It seems that the information concerning the danger of live vaccines in some children is not being delivered to the doctors for them to inform their parents. This is valuable information. Will Avery develop MS in the future? Is this vaccine going to be the "trigger?"

I believe that undiagnosed Celiac Disease, in combination with increased vaccine requirements, is creating increases in autism, MS, ADHD, and other autoimmune diseases.

Shouldn't doctors test children for the gene for Celiac Disease before they recommend them getting a vaccine that may not be good for them? Shouldn't the doctors listen when a parent tells them about a family history that may predispose the child to complications from the vaccine?

I believe we should try to PREVENT as many cases of autism, MS, and other autoimmune diseases as we can.

Quoting Barry Segal, founder and president of Focus for Health, "The vaccine question is not a simple 'for' or 'against' issue. Vaccination is necessary, but it is a given that vaccination causes adverse events in some recipients. It makes sense, then, that children with a history of earaches, gut problems, skin rashes, etc., should be treated with more precaution, as potentially vulnerable, and be vaccinated differently."

Can a gluten-free diet help children with autism? Can they be cured?

According to the autism website Tacanow.org, "The GFCF (gluten-free, casein-free) diet helps 91% of the autistic children out there in improving everything about their learning disabilities and overall well-being. This includes better speech, better bowel movements than before, better sleep patterns, less cranky behaviors, less stimmy behaviors (stimmy is short for "self-stimulation" and is a term used to describe self-stimulating behaviors such as rocking, spinning, hand flapping, etc.), less foggy/dazed looks, and more ready to learn that ever before."

Recovery from autism is real!

DEBBIE MCGRANN

ABUNDANCE

"The first wealth is health."
Ralph Waldo Emerson

HEALTHY

Enjoying health and vigor of body, mind, or spirit.

WEALTHY

Having an abundance of material possessions, resources, or money.

WISE

Characterized by wisdom (insight, good sense, judgment). Marked by deep understanding, keen discernment and a capacity for sound judgment.

CHAPTER TWELVE

Living Life to Its Fullest

Healthy, Wealthy & Wise

A new year! I was starting my first full year of recovery. What was next? I sold the business that I no longer wanted to do. Then, it was my time to start something new. I decided to become a real estate agent. I reasoned that I still needed to be in charge of my time, so I could not have a regular 9-5 job. As a real estate agent, I would be in control of when I would show properties and do other activities with clients. It was something I had always wanted to do.

I had enough stamina to take the 9-3 classes four days a week for two weeks. I was able to pass the state required test on the first try! I am grateful that my life had changed for the better since my diagnosis. I chose real estate because I had invested in real estate and understood how good it was for people to own real estate. I enjoyed helping home buyers start to create family wealth through home ownership.

As I noted earlier, my first year with Coldwell Banker, resulted in my being named "Rookie of the Year" (not bad for a recovered MS patient)!

Also, I needed my freedom. At the beginning of my recovery, I still needed a lot of rest. I had gotten stronger, but still had some health issues that might not go away. A 9-5 job was not a good idea. I did not want to have the stress of asking for special accommodations on the job. Also, I wanted to be my own boss, and not have my income limited by a regular job.

My first grandchild was born March 10, 2009. I was healthy enough to stay a week in North Carolina helping my daughter and son-in-law with baby Ella. I spent my first birthday since my recovery, March 17, in North Carolina. I was so grateful that day. I remembered that, a year before, I had been reluctant to hold the newborn baby, Patrick, at his baptism party. I had come so far!

I have shared my health journey with you and many other people with the hope that my story of recovery from Multiple Sclerosis will help someone. As a result, many people have contacted me to share their own story of recovery. Also, many wanted more information and encouragement.

I celebrate my recovery every Mother's Day! I am symptom free and getting stronger every day. I follow the gluten-free diet and get plenty of rest and sunshine. And I am still drug-free! My sister and I celebrated my 60th birthday (and her 50th) March 17, 2014 by going to Disney World for a gluten-free tea, quite an accomplishment. We had doubted I would reach my 60th birthday!

After recovering from Multiple Sclerosis, I am able to pursue a career as a real estate salesperson with Coldwell Banker. My disability gives me insight into the needs of buyers and sellers with disabilities. I am committed to helping people with disabilities achieve home ownership. How can I help you?

"The first wealth is health."
Ralph Waldo Emerson

As Emerson says, "The first wealth is health." When you are not in good health, everything else in your life is harder. When you are in pain or ill, it is harder to be a good parent, spouse, friend, or employee. And your relationships with everyone may be strained.

Have you ever heard the expression, trust your gut instinct? That means fortitude and stamina in coping with what alarms, repels, or discourages. Some scientists are now linking gut health with decision making. I know from experience that you should never make important decisions when you are not well!

When my symptoms started getting worse, I was afraid that my family finances were going to suffer. In preparation for the future, I sought advice from a financial planner. I had met her at a business networking group. I met with her and her partner in their office. I explained to both of them that my disability was increasing, and that I was not confident that I would be able to work much longer. Her partner went over all the financial information that I had provided. He assured me that my husband and I had done well saving for our retirement, and, at our ages of 49 and 47, we could expect a comfortable early retirement if necessary. I left feeling relieved.

The next day, I received a phone call from the financial planner. She asked if I would like to meet her for lunch because she had some follow-up information for me. I agreed. When she arrived, she started telling me how her partner John was not taking me seriously because I was a woman. She said she had had that problem frequently. She told me that she had a better investment for me – one that John had not told me about because he didn't think women were smart enough to understand the benefits of this type of investment. She was very convincing. My gut instinct was trying to tell me that this was a bad idea. The warning signs were there. A financial adviser should not meet you outside the office and speak badly about another adviser. However, I was very sick and desperate for help. I agreed to the investment and gave her the money.

I regretted it immediately. She was a fraud. It didn't take long for me to realize my mistake. I called her office to talk to her about ending our relationship. I was told that she had left the company. I asked to speak to her supervisor, and told him what had happened. He stopped taking my calls.

I had no option but to sue her company to get my money back. I was so embarrassed when I told the lawyer what happened. He reassured me that she was a very convincing fraud. He told me I was not the only person that she had done this to. He told me there was a well-known lawyer who was a victim of her scheme, too. I was able to recover some of my money, but not all of it. My trust was shattered. I had come to her for help as a disabled person who was getting worse, and she took advantage of me. Take my advice, if you need help financially, be careful who you trust. Talk to your family and friends so they can recommend someone. Take someone with you to help with the details. Take your time making your decision. Trust but verify.

Wealthy

Poverty can be the perfect teacher for people who want to be wealthy. Poverty teaches you what you want in life and what you don't want. My parents learned early in life what they did not want their lives to look like. They both came from poverty and they did not want to stay there or to return. However, they also learned that, in most cases, poverty is not fatal. When they were children living in poverty, there was no welfare, no food stamps, no free school lunches, or any of the social programs that we now have available for families struggling with poverty. They grew up in rented homes with no heat, no electricity, and, in my mother's case, no indoor plumbing. These were tough lessons to learn, but they learned those lessons and used them to help shape their successful future.

I think my parents married as teenagers to escape their difficult family situations. I think they thought that if they worked together, they could better their lives. I often wonder if they had a plan and goals, or did they just throw caution into the wind. I suspect that they had no plan. Remember the times they lived in: They had experienced the Great Depression, the devastation of the Dust Bowl, and World War II in Washington DC. My mother had survived a severe accident. I think these experiences gave them the courage to start living on their own at a very young age, but they wanted to do it together. They married in 1952. My brother was born in 1953 and I was born in 1954. My sister was born in 1964 when things were different in our family.

My grandmother's goal of home ownership was shared by my mother and father. Their first goal was to own their first home. My mother did have a plan for this goal. She started her family's wealth creation with a dime. She decided she would save enough dimes for the down payment on their home. Every day when my father returned home from working (he worked three jobs), she would take all the dimes from his pockets and add them to her savings. She shared her plan with my grandmother; and I'm sure my grandmother gave her as many dimes, as she could spare. Shortly, she had reached her goal of $1,500 in dimes and they owned their first home. She was still a teenager and my father was barely in his 20's with two children under two. It was tough, but she did it. As they say, "When the going gets tough, the tough get going."

My parents' next goal was to own a rental property. Within five years of buying their first house, my parents bought the house next door. These houses were very modest houses in a low-income neighborhood. Our family moved into the new house, and we rented the house next door. Shortly after that move, my parents bought another modest house, less than 1,000 square feet, in the same neighborhood. Then, our family moved into that house. Within ten years, my parents owned their own home and two rental properties. They were both under 30 years of age - not bad for two kids coming out of poverty. And it all started with a dime!

My mother and father started to build wealth for their family with a dime and a goal of home ownership - the American Dream! When my mother died suddenly at the age of 69, she and my father had accumulated an estate of over $1,000,000.00 in assets. They grew their wealth slowly and steadily by investing in rental properties, stocks, bonds, and saving their money. They always lived in modest homes. They were most proud of having provided affordable, clean, and safe housing to over 20 families.

By the way, start saving your dimes; it's still possible to buy a house with only $1,500. I can show you how to start accumulating wealth for your family by buying your own home, and then buying rental properties. My family did it, and so can yours.

debbie@theaccidentalcure.com

Wise

"Pain can change you, but that doesn't mean it has to be a bad change. Take that pain and turn it into wisdom."
The Dalai Lama

Wisdom comes from a culmination of our life experiences - good and bad. I think that the lessons we learn from our mistakes and our successes are far more impactful than knowledge learned in academia. If we become lifetime learners, we will strengthen our ability to be self-reliant and resilient.

Listen to the stories of your family's successes and what they describe as their failures. Is there really such a thing as failure? I believe in what Thomas Edison said about his "failed" experiments:

"I have not failed. I've just found 10,000 ways that won't work."

My father taught my brother, my sister, and me that success leaves clues. He told us to pay attention to the people in our community who were successful and follow the example of what they do. He told us to study successful people and learn from their success and failures.

Wisdom from our pain is not soon forgotten. Pain leaves scars, but it also leaves important lessons and increased emotional strength. I had to grieve for the pain of the loss of my time. I had to forgive myself for the pain of financial loss. I learned from my physical pain that I was tougher than I thought. Now I have the confidence to take on new things. That's wisdom! Remember, what doesn't kill you makes you stronger!

"If you are not your own doctor, you are a fool."
Hippocrates

The "What If" Mantra

After going through the most difficult health experience of my life, I started to think what I call the "What If" thinking game. The "What If" game questions whether Celiac Disease is the root of all evil when it comes to autoimmune diseases. I am confident from my research that if we observe and investigate our unique situation with respect to diagnoses of diseases that come with a life sentence, and very little hope of improvement; we may discover that we simply have a disease that has been misdiagnosed or missing the critical link to Celiac Disease. It is well documented in the medical community that a patient with one autoimmune disease is likely to have or develop another autoimmune disease. Why? I believe we need to look to a relationship to Celiac Disease as the root cause of multiple autoimmune diseases.

WHAT IF?

What if Multiple Sclerosis is a symptom of Celiac Disease? What if Celiac Disease is the root of all evil of MS and other autoimmune diseases? That would be wonderful news! The only treatment for Celiac Disease is a lifelong gluten-free diet. This explains why my MS symptoms disappeared when I started my gluten-free diet.

WHAT IF?

What if <u>Alzheimer's & Dementia are symptoms</u> of Celiac Disease?

What if <u>Attention Deficit Hyperactivity Disorder (ADHD) is a symptom</u> of Celiac Disease?

What if <u>Arthritis is a symptom</u> of Celiac Disease?

What if <u>Asthma is a symptom</u> of Celiac Disease?

What if <u>Autism is a symptom</u> of Celiac Disease?

What if <u>Cancer is a symptom</u> of Celiac Disease?

What if <u>Colitis & IBD are symptoms</u> of Celiac Disease?

What if <u>Crohn's Disease is a symptom</u> of Celiac Disease?

What if <u>Depression & Mental Illness are symptoms</u> of Celiac Disease?

What if <u>Diabetes is a symptom</u> of Celiac Disease?

What if <u>Epilepsy is a symptom</u> of Celiac Disease?

What if <u>Fibromyalgia is a symptom</u> of Celiac Disease?

What if <u>Infertility & Miscarriage are symptoms</u> of Celiac Disease?

What if <u>Liver Disease is a symptom</u> of Celiac Disease?

What if <u>Lupus is a symptom</u> of Celiac Disease?

What if <u>Lymphoma is a symptom</u> of Celiac Disease?

What if <u>Migraines are a symptom</u> of Celiac Disease?

What if <u>Multiple Sclerosis is a symptom</u> of Celiac Disease?

What if <u>Osteoporosis is a symptom</u> of Celiac Disease?

What if <u>Psoriasis & Eczema are symptoms</u> of Celiac Disease?

Saving Billions of Dollars and Lives by Diet

Celiac Disease **CAUSED** my **MS**, therefore, the gluten-free diet, **CURED** my **MS**. Could it be that simple? For me and thousands like me, it is. The fact that I never took any drugs for my MS is proof that it was diet alone that saved me. Imagine all of the patients who were suffering from other autoimmune diseases who would be helped with a gluten-free diet.

How many billions of dollars would the health insurance companies and families save if we did not need all of the drugs? How many lives would be saved from the deadly side effects of these drugs?

Are you that patient? I would encourage anyone who has been diagnosed with an autoimmune disease, or who has unexplained symptoms, to start a gluten-free diet immediately, before starting any drug treatment. If you do the diet before drug therapy, the doctors can't claim that the drugs made you better and not the diet. The diet won't hurt you and will likely help you. The drugs could kill you.

There are NO drugs available for treating Celiac Disease. Thank God! Maintaining a gluten-free diet without a diagnosis of Celiac Disease has enjoyed widespread acceptance. We don't need our doctor's permission to help ourselves get better. We must be our own doctor. Remember, if it is going to be, it is up to us.

List of 100 Autoimmune Diseases

According to the American Autoimmune Related Diseases Association, there are over 100 known autoimmune diseases. I have mentioned only a few. Autoimmune diseases are hard to diagnose; it may take up to three years to get a proper diagnosis. Autoimmune diseases affect women far more often than men: 75% of Americans with autoimmune disease are women. As an example, 9 out of 10 people who have lupus are women. (1) The annual financial burden is estimated to be over $100 billion dollars in direct health costs.

What if most of these autoimmune diseases could be managed by a gluten-free diet? The financial savings would be incredible. In addition, the restoration of health to all these patients would be priceless!

Achalasia
Addison's disease
Adult Still's disease
Agammaglobulinemia
Alopecia areata
Amyloidosis
Ankylosing spondylitis
Anti-GBM/Anti-TBM nephritis
Antiphospholipid syndrome Autoimmune angioedema
Autoimmune dysautonomia
Autoimmune encephalomyelitis
Autoimmune hepatitis
Autoimmune inner ear disease (AIED)
Autoimmune myocarditis
Autoimmune oophoritis
Autoimmune orchitis
Autoimmune pancreatitis
Autoimmune retinopathy

Autoimmune urticaria
Axonal & neuronal neuropathy (AMAN)
Baló disease
Behcet's disease
Benign mucosal pemphigoid
Bullous pemphigoid
Castleman disease (CD)
Celiac disease
Chagas disease
Chronic inflammatory demyelinating polyneuropathy (CIDP)
Chronic recurrent multifocal osteomyelitis (CRMO)
Churg-Strauss Syndrome (CSS) or Eosinophilic Granulomatosis (EGPA)
Cicatricial pemphigoid
Cogan's syndrome
Cold agglutinin disease
Congenital heart block Coxsackie myocarditis
CREST syndrome
Crohn's disease
Dermatitis herpetiformis
Dermatomyositis
Devic's disease (neuromyelitis optica)
Discoid lupus
Dressler's syndrome
Endometriosis
Eosinophilic esophagitis (EoE)
Eosinophilic fasciitis Erythema nodosum
Essential mixed cryoglobulinemia
Evans syndrome
Fibromyalgia
Fibrosing alveolitis
Giant cell arteritis (temporal arteritis)
Giant cell myocarditis
Glomerulonephritis
Goodpasture's syndrome
Granulomatosis with Polyangiitis
Graves' disease

Guillain-Barre syndrome
Hashimoto's thyroiditis
Hemolytic anemia
Henoch-Schonlein purpura (HSP)
Herpes gestationis or pemphigoid gestationis (PG)
Hidradenitis Suppurativa (HS) (Acne Inversa)
Hypogammalglobulinemia
IgA Nephropathy
IgG4-related sclerosing disease
Immune thrombocytopenic purpura (ITP)
Inclusion body myositis (IBM)
Interstitial cystitis (IC)
Juvenile arthritis
Juvenile diabetes (Type 1 diabetes)
Juvenile myositis (JM)
Kawasaki disease
Lambert-Eaton syndrome
Leukocytoclastic vasculitis
Lichen planus
Lichen sclerosus
Ligneous conjunctivitis
Linear IgA disease (LAD)
Lupus
Lyme disease chronic
Meniere's disease
Microscopic polyangiitis (MPA)
Mixed connective tissue disease (MCTD)
Mooren's ulcer
Mucha-Habermann disease
Multifocal Motor Neuropathy (MMN) or MMNCB
Multiple sclerosis
Myasthenia gravis
Myositis
Narcolepsy
Neonatal Lupus
Neuromyelitis optica
Neutropenia
Ocular cicatricial pemphigoid
Optic neuritis

Palindromic rheumatism (PR)
PANDAS
Paraneoplastic cerebellar degeneration (PCD)
Paroxysmal nocturnal hemoglobinuria (PNH)
Parry Romberg syndrome
Pars planitis (peripheral uveitis)
Parsonage-Turner syndrome
Pemphigus
Peripheral neuropathy
Perivenous encephalomyelitis
Pernicious anemia (PA)
POEMS syndrome
Polyarteritis nodosa
Polyglandular syndromes type I, II, III
Polymyalgia rheumatica
Polymyositis
Postmyocardial infarction syndrome
Postpericardiotomy syndrome
Primary biliary cirrhosis
Primary sclerosing cholangitis
Progesterone dermatitis
Psoriasis
Psoriatic arthritis
Pure red cell aplasia (PRCA)
Pyoderma gangrenosum
Raynaud's phenomenon
Reactive Arthritis
Reflex sympathetic dystrophy Relapsing polychondritis
Restless legs syndrome (RLS)
Retroperitoneal fibrosis
Rheumatic fever
Rheumatoid arthritis
Sarcoidosis
Schmidt syndrome
Scleritis
Scleroderma
Sjögren's syndrome
Sperm & testicular autoimmunity
Stiff person syndrome (SPS)

Subacute bacterial endocarditis (SBE)
Susac's syndrome
Sympathetic ophthalmia (SO)
Takayasu's arteritis
Temporal arteritis/Giant cell arteritis
Thrombocytopenic purpura (TTP)
Tolosa-Hunt syndrome (THS)
Transverse myelitis
Type 1 diabetes
Ulcerative colitis (UC)
Undifferentiated connective tissue disease (UCTD)
Uveitis
Vasculitis
Vitiligo
Vogt-Koyanagi-Harada Disease

(1) National Women's Health Information Center, U.S. Department of Health and Human Services, Office on Women's Health. WomensHealth.gov/faq/lupus/pdf

DEBBIE MCGRANN

*"Have you ever heard the statement, "If I can do it, so can you?" It gives you hope, doesn't it?
But it's not the complete story.
It should say, "If I can do it, so can you, IF you do what I did."*

Zig Ziglar

THE ACCIDENTAL CURE

EPILOGUE

Lessons Learned

Despite my personal challenges to date, I feel absolutely wonderful! I believe that I was guided to my cure by divine connections that seemed accidental at the time. I was given this task to help others, and I want to reach out to as many people as possible and tell them my story. I consider myself a change agent. I am now confident in my ability to help others with their health questions.

Unfortunately, my doctors were not successful in helping me navigate through my illness to my cure. Initially, I was the type of person who always listened to the opinion of the doctors and other professionals. Not anymore! I think that their focus needs to change in order to see greater success in the lives of others. For example, they are putting profits ahead of their patients' health. The pharmaceutical industry has created a revenue stream, and doctors are caught up in the web. They are narrow-minded in some cases, and the medical fields are too specialized. I will never again question my ability to solve problems, no matter how difficult. I have learned to never trust someone's opinion more than mine. I have learned to believe in myself more than ever.

I believe that the pharmaceutical industry must make changes as well. The pharmaceutical industry is now more aggressive and powerful. The law allowing them to advertise may have created these problems. They are creating diseases to match the drugs that they have (consider acid reflux and the purple pill). In addition, they created the opioid crisis that is destroying families and killing thousands.

My Personal Recommendations

1. Don't rely on the doctors for all of your information. Do your own research. However, stay on official medical websites. There is a lot of false information on the internet.

2. Share your story. You never know from where important information will come. I received hints from casual conversations.

3. Look for hints in your family. What illnesses are common?

4. This is probably the most important: have faith in yourself and your ability to be in control of your health decisions. If I had followed the advice of one of my doctors, I would be dead now. Trust but verify. Research the advice that your doctors give you. You don't have to do what they say!

5. Take charge, ask questions, and be curious.

The insurance companies should protect their clients' health by restricting access to these deadly drugs and their many side effects (some of which are worse than the original disease). What if the insurance companies required patients diagnosed with any autoimmune disease to try the gluten-free diet treatment before the drugs? The insurance companies would save BILLIONS of dollars!

And, the patients might have much better outcomes. "At first, do no harm"! They could provide nutritional guidance and gluten-free food with all of the money they would save.

What if there was an inexpensive and safe way to screen MS patients and others before the drugs were started? I have heard of a medical device that can be swallowed. It is the size of a vitamin capsule. It contains a camera with resolution strong enough to see the damaged villi that causes malabsorption and that caused my MS. This device is projected to cost only $500!

This screening may also help prevent autism by screening children before they are vaccinated, and the damage is done. Prevention is much cheaper and much safer than treating a disease.

Doctors should have more training in non-drug solutions. The drug companies should be limited in their contact and compensation to doctors. Drugs should not be a revenue stream for doctors. Doctors should encourage their patients to think of wellness as their responsibility. There should be more emphasis on nutrition as a solution to diseases. Patients with chronic illnesses need more time with a doctor/nurse/nutritionist because these are complex issues. The solutions do not have to be expensive, dangerous drugs.

We need to tell autoimmune patients that there could be a link to Celiac Disease, and they should go on a gluten-free diet to see if they feel better. If they feel better, they should assume they have Celiac Disease and stay on the gluten-free diet. It won't hurt, unlike the drugs.

> "First, do no harm"
> Hippocratic Oath

References

This guide is a small sample of the information that is available concerning celiac disease and other autoimmune diseases. Since there are over 100 autoimmune diseases, it was impossible to include all the current information for each autoimmune disease. Please visit our website, www.theaccidentalcure.com to access the information sighted here, and for additional information as we continue our research.

ADD and ADHD
Adelman, T., & Behrend, J. (2000). *Special Foods for Special Kids. Practical Solutions & Great Recipes for Children with Food Allergies.* Brandon, Or: Robert Reed Publishers.

Gottschall, E. (1994). Breaking the Vicious Disease. *Journal of Attention Disorders.* 10 (2), 200-204.

Gungor, S., et.al. (2013) Frequency of celiac disease in attention-deficit/hyperactivity disorder. *Journal of Pediatric Gastroenterology and Nutrition. 56* (2), 211-214.

Niederhofer, H., & Pittschieler, K. (2006). A preliminary investigation of ADHD symptoms in persons with celiac disease. *Journal of Attention Disorders. 10* (2): 200-204.

Alzheimer's and Dementia
Lurie, Y., et al. (2008) Celiac disease diagnosed in the elderly. *Journal of Clinical Gastoenterol, 42* (1), 59-61.

Makhlouf, S., et al. (2018). Cognitive impairment in celiac disease and non-celiac gluten sensitivity: Review of literature on the main cognitive impairments, the imaging and the effect of gluten free diet.
Acta Neurologica Belgica, 118 (1), *21-27.*

Arthritis
Atteno, M., et al. (2013). The occurrence of lower limb enthesopathy in

coeliac disease patients without clinical signs of articular involvement. *Rheumatology*, 52(5), 893-897.

Podas, T., et al. (2007). Is rheumatoid arthritis a disease that starts in the intestine? A pilot study comparing an element diet with oral prednisolone. *Postgraduate Medical Journal, 83* (976), 128-131.

Asthma
Kero, J., et. al. (2001). Could TH1 and TH2 diseases coexist? Evaluation of asthma incidence in children with coeliac disease, type 1 diabetes, or rheumatoid arthritis: A register study. *The Journal of Allergy and Clinical Immunology, 108* (5) 781-783.

Ludvigsson, J. F., et al. (2011). Celiac disease confers a 1.6 – fold increased risk of asthma. A nationwide population-based cohort study. *The Journal of Allergy and Clinical Immunology, 127* (4), 1071-1073.

Autism
Calderoni, S., et al. (2016). Serological screening for celiac disease in 382 pre-schoolers with Autism Spectrum Disorder. *Italian Journal of Pediatrics, 42*(1), 98.

Jepson, B. (2007). *Changing the Course of Autism: A Scientific Approach for Parents and Physicians.* Boulder, CO: First Sentient Publications.

Lewis, L. (1998). *Special Diets for Special Kids: Understanding and Implementing Special Diets to Aid in the Treatment of Autism and Related Developmental Disorders.* Arlington, TX: Future Horizons, Inc.

Ludvigsson, J. F. et. al. (2013). A nationwide study of the association between celiac disease and the risk of autistic spectrum disorders. *JAMA Psychiatry, 70*(11), 1224-1230.

McCarthy, J. (2007). *Louder than Words: A Mother's Journey in Healing Autism.* New York, NY: Penguin Books, Ltd.

Seroussi, K. (2014). *Unraveling the Mystery of Autism and Pervasive Developmental Disorder.* New York, NY: Simon and Shuster.

Autoimmune Disease

Fasano, A., & Shea-Donohue, T. (2005) Mechanisms of disease: The role of intestinal barrier function in the pathogenesis of gastrointestinal autoimmune diseases. *Nature Clinical Practice Gastroenteroly and Hepatology,* 2(9) 416-422.

Lerner, A., & Matthias, T. (2015). Changes in intestinal tight junction permeability associated with industrial food additives explain the rising incidence of autoimmune disease. *Autoimmunity Reviews, 14* (6), 479-489.

Cancer

Fasano, A. (2011) Zonulin and its regulation of intestinal barrier function: The biological door to inflammation, autoimmunity, and cancer. *Physiological Reviews, 91*(1), 151-175.

Celiac Disease

Fasano, A. (2009) Surprises from celiac disease. *Scientific American. 301*(2), 54-61.

Colitis and Irritable Bowel Syndrome

Gottschall, E. (1994). *Breaking the Vicious Cycle: Intestinal Health through Diet.* Ontario, Canada: Kirkton Press.

Herfarth, H.H., et al. (2014). Prevalence of a gluten-free diet and improvement of clinical symptoms in patients with inflammatory bowel diseases. *Inflammatory Bowel Disease. 20* (7), 1194-1197

Matteoni, C. A., et al. (2001) Celiac disease is highly prevalent in lymphocytic colitis. *Journal of Clinical Gastroenterology, 32* (3), 225-227.

Zwolinska-Wcislo, M., et al. (2009). Frequency of celiac disease and irritable bowel syndrome coexistance and its influence on the disease course. *Przeglad Lekarski, 66*(3) 126-129. (Article in Polish).

Crohn's
Lail, G., et al. (2016) Coexistence of celiac and crohn's disease in a patient presenting with chronic diarrhea. *J Coll Physicians Surg Pak, 26* (6), 536-538.

Depression
Busby, E., et al. (2018). Mood disorders and gluten: It's not all in your mind! A systematic review with meta-analysis. *Nutrients, 10* (11) pii : 1708. doi:10.3390/nu10111708.

Diabetes
Serena, G., et. al. (2015). The role of gluten in celiac disease and type 1 diabetes. *Journal of Nutrients, 7 (9)*, 7143-7162.

Simmons, J.H., et. al. (2011). Celiac autoimmunity in children with type 1 diabetes: A two-year follow-up. *The Journal of Pediatrics, 158* (2), 276-281.

Diet
Afshin, A., et al. (2019). *Health effects of dietary risks in 195 countries, 1990-2017: A systematic analysis for the Global Burden of Disease Study 2017. Lancet, 393* (10184), 1958-1972.

Madzhidova, S., & Sedrakyan, L. (2019). The use of dietary interventions in pediatric patients. *Pharmacy, 7*(10), 1-13.
Consumer Dummies. (2015). *Gluten-free for Dummies.* Hoboken, NJ: John Wiley & Sons.

Drugs
Sturgeon, C., & Fasano, A. (2016). Zonulin, a regulator of epithelial and endothelial barrier functions, and its involvement in chronic inflammatory diseases. *Tissue Barriers, 4(4).doi:10.1080/21688370.2016.1251384.*

Pruimboom, L. & de Punder, K. (2015). The opioid effects of gluten exorphins: asymptomatic celiac disease. *Journal of Health, Population, and Nutrition, 33(24), and following.*

Epilepsy
Ludvigsson, J.F. et. al. (2012). Increased risk of epilepsy in biopsy-verified celiac disease: a population-based cohort study. *Neurology*, 78 (18), 14011407.

Fibromyalgia
Isasi, C., et al. (2014). Fibromyalgia and non-celiac gluten sensitivity: A description with remission of fibromyalgia. *Rheumatology International*, 34(11), 1607-1612.doi: 10.1007/s00296-014-2990-6.

Gluten-Free Diet
Bhatia, B. K., et. al. *(2014). Diet and psoriasis, part II:* Celiac disease and role of a gluten-free diet. *Journal of the American Academy of Dermatology*, 71(2), 350-358.

Kasarda, D.D. (2013). Can an increase in celiac disease be attributed to an increase in the gluten content of wheat as a consequence of wheat breeding. *Journal of Agricultural and Food Chemistry, 61 (6), 1155-1159*

Sapone, A., et al. (2012). Spectrum of gluten-related disorders: consensus on new nomenclature and Classification. *BMC Medicine, 10* (13) and following.

Infertility and Miscarriage
Choi, J.M., et al. (2011). Increased prevalence of celiac disease in patients with unexplained infertility in the United States: A prospective study. *The Journal of Reproductive Medicine*, 56 (5-6), 199-203.

Liver
Zali, M.R., et al. (2011). Liver complications in celiac disease. *Hepatitis Monthly,11*(5), 333-341.

Lupus
Ludvigsson, J.F., et al. (2012). Increased Risk of Systemic Lupus Erythematosus in 29,000 Patients with Biopsy-verified Celiac Disease. *The Journal of Rheumatology*, 39(10), 1964-1970.

Lymphoma
Catassi, C., et al. (2002). Risk of non-Hodgkin lymphoma in celiac disease. *JAMA, 287* (11), 1413-1419.

Mental Illness
Bressan, P., & Kramer, P. (2016) Bread and other edibles agents of mental disease. *Frontiers in Human Neuroscience, 10* 130 and following.

Jackson, J.R., et al. (2012). Neurologic and psychiatric manifestations of celiac disease and gluten sensitivity. *The Psychiatric Quarterly, 83* (1), 91102.

Levinta, A., et. al. (2018). Use of a gluten-free diet in schizophrenia: A systematic review. Advances in Nutrition, *9*(6), 824-832.

Migraines
Ameghino, L., et al. (2019) Headache in patients with celiac disease and its response to the gluten-free diet. *Journal of Oral & Facial Pain and Headache, 33*(3), 294-300.

Zis, P., et al. (2018). Headache associated with coeliac disease: A systematic review and meta-analysis. *Nutrients, 10*(10), 445 and following.

Multiple Sclerosis
Sawyer, A., & Bachrack. J. (2007). *The MS Recovery Diet: Take Control of Your Health, Change What You Eat, and Live Symptom-Free.* New York, NY: Penguin Group.

Osteoporosis
Holick, M. (2012*). The Vitamin D Solution: A 3-Step Strategy to Cure Our Most Common Health Problems*. Indianapolis, Indiana, IN: Wiley Publishing

Krums, L., et al. (2018). Reproductive disorders, osteoporosis and secondary hyperparathyroidism with celiac disease. *Teraperticheskii arkhiv, 90*(10), 89-93.

Psoriasis and Eczema

Bhatia, B.K., et al. (2014) Diet and psoriasis, part II: celiac disease and role of a gluten-free diet. *Journal of the American Academy of Dermatology,71*(2), 350-358.

Ciacci, C., et al. (2015). The gluten-free diet and its current application in coeliac disease and dermatitis herpetiformis. *United European Gastroenterology Journal, 3*(2), 121-135.

Vaccinations

Anania, C. et al. (2017). Immune response to vaccines in children with celiac disease. *World Journal of Gastroenterology 23* (18), 3205-3213.

Opri, R., et al. (2015). Immune response to hepatitis B vaccine in patients with celiac disease: A systematic review and meta-analysis. *Human Vaccines & Immunotherapeutics 11*(12): 2800-2805.

Rostami, K., & Nejad, M.R. (2013). Vaccinations in celiac disease. *Journal of Pediatric Gastroenterology and Nutrition, 56*(4), 341-342.

Centers for Disease Control and Prevention. (1993). Recommendations of the Advisory Committee on Immunization Practices (AZIP): Use of Vaccines and Immune Globulins in Persons with Altered Immunocompetence. *MMWR* (42), (No. RR-4): {inclusive page numbers}.

Additional References

Hill, N. (2003). *Think and Grow Rich*. New York, NY: Penguin Group.

Osteen, J. (2004). *Your Best Life Now: 7 Steps to Living AT Your Full Potential*. New York, NY: FaithWords Publishing.

Peale, N. (1952). *The Power of Positive Thinking*. New York, NY: Prentice Hall.

Shuller, R. (1984). *Tough Times Never Last, But Tough People Do!* New York, NY: Bantam

Shuller, R. (1997). *If It is Going to Be, It's Up to Me: The Eight Proven Principles of Possibility Thinking*. New York, NY: HarperCollins Publishers.

Trezise, K., & Power, J. *(2015). My Journey to an Organized Life : A Creative Road Map for Organizing Your Time, Space, and Finances*. North Charleston, SC: Create Space.

Embry, A. (2012). *The Tysabri Debacle*. Retrieved March 24, 2012, from http://www.direct-ms.org/
National Women's Health Information Center, U.S. Department of Health and Human Services, Office on Women's Health. WomensHealth.gov/faq/lupus/pdf

THE ACCIDENTAL CURE

"When you give someone a book, you don't give him just paper, ink, and glue. You give him the possibility of a whole new life."
Christopher Morley

Who Can You Help?

By writing this book and telling my story, it is my wish that I have filled you with hope — hope that you can be well again. Hope that you can mend strained relationships caused by your illness. Hope for a better financial future. The ripple effect of helping others can be enormous.

If you have found hope and value in what you have learned in this book, consider giving a copy to people about whom you care, and who you think need the information that I have provided to improve their lives. My goal is to bring awareness of Celiac Disease and its devastating effects on our health. Who do you know who needs this information?

This book could bring better health to your family, friends, coworkers, or a stranger who has shared their story of ill health with you. Like me, they may not know that there is a way for them to get better safely! Please help me pay this forward. Thank you! List people who would benefit from this book.

1) _____

2) _____

3) _____

4) _____

5) _____

Speaking Engagements

Debbie McGrann is a passionate speaker and trusted advisor to people suffering from chronic autoimmune diseases and other disabilities. As an entrepreneur with a chronic illness, she provides valuable insight for corporations and organizations that strive to develop the healthiest workplace.

Debbie empowers her audiences with confidence to think for themselves, ask questions, and seek answers. Her presentations motivate people to pursue the knowledge that will help them recover and live richer, more rewarding lives. Debbie's approach is always one of compassionate professionalism with an appropriate dose of humor!

All programs, from keynote speeches to in-house seminars, are customized to maximize your attendees' experience.

To book Debbie McGrann for your next conference or in-house event, please contact at debbie@theaccidentalcure.com

ORGANIZATIONS and CORPORATIONS

This book is available at special quantity discounts for bulk purchases. This book is perfect for employee gifts, sales promotions, premiums, or fund-raising. Give the gift of health!

For information contact:

debbie@theaccidentalcure.com

Thank you!

About the Author

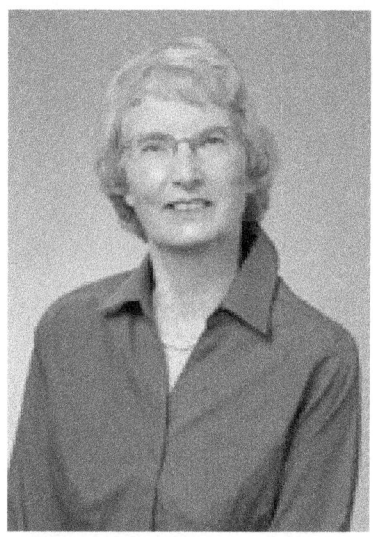

When a break-through solution to a serious health condition is discovered, it should be shared with the world. That is precisely what Debbie McGrann is doing with this publication of *The Accidental Cure*. Who would have thought that a layperson, who discarded the advice of her so-called expert physicians, could discover a cure for her alarming and frightening declining health!

In this book, Debbie shares the story of her journey to good health so that the hundreds (perhaps thousands!) with Multiple Sclerosis (MS)/Celiac Disease, or any of the more than 100 known autoimmune disorders, can benefit from her research. She empathizes with those who are terrified about possibly dying too soon – especially in view of their physicians who either explicitly say that they can offer no help, or who only have a prescription drug that Debbie's research has discovered had the very real possibility of causing death!

Debbie hopes and prays that if you know someone with MS, or any of the 100 known autoimmune diseases, or with symptoms that sound like they could indicate MS, you will share this book with them. Of course, be aware that not everyone who has MS or Celiac Disease will have the same set of symptoms as she had.

Debbie's writing style is both engaging and entertaining. You likely will find it hard to put down until you reach the very last page!

www.ingramcontent.com/pod-product-compliance
Lightning Source LLC
Chambersburg PA
CBHW032046150426
43194CB00006B/442